The
Good Gut
Guide

Help for IBS • Ulcerative Colitis
Crohn's Disease • Diverticulitis
Food Allergies • Other Gut Problems

Stephanie Zinser

Foreword by Professor R. John Nicholls

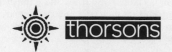

Thorsons
An Imprint of HarperCollins*Publishers*
77–85 Fulham Palace Road,
Hammersmith, London W6 8JB

The website address is: www.thorsonselement.com

and *Thorsons* are trademarks of
HarperCollins*Publishers* Ltd

First published by Thorsons 2003

1 3 5 7 9 10 8 6 4 2

A catalogue record of this book is
available from the British Library

ISBN 0 00 713805 9

Printed and bound in Great Britain by
Creative Print & Design (Wales), Ebbw Vale

Contents

SECTION 3

Acknowledgements

Very few books are written without help. This is no exception.

I am deeply indebted to Dr Stuart Gould who, despite having looked after me through my worst years of illness, was still willing to spend long hours helping me with many of the medical aspects of this book. I am also indebted to Professor John Nicholls, who carried out the surgery which cured me of my illness and who kindly agreed to pen the foreword. Grateful thanks go to several experts for their technical help: Professors Glenn R Gibson, John Hermon-Taylor, John Cummings, Derek Jewell and Nick Read; and Dr John Hunter, Penny Nunn and Tracey Virgin-Elliston.

I would also like to thank the following: Rory Clements for giving me my first chance in journalism; Bonnie Estridge for persuading me to write this book; Grant Feller for providing sound advice and lots of work; Marie Pay for her brilliant suggestions; and Andrea Scott and Elaine Maxwell-Muller for looking after my family so well while I was writing this book. I am also grateful to all those who generously shared their own stories – and to Wanda Whiteley for being such a positive and enthusiastic editor.

Finally, thank you to my three children Emily, Jenny and Katie, my husband Steve and my parents for being an endless source of love, understanding and encouragement.

Foreword

In the last 20 years an increasingly informed public has acquired considerable medical knowledge. This has come through printed media, television and the Internet – and by contact with health care professionals like doctors and nurses.

People working in medicine who understand the need for greater communication often find this terribly rewarding. Taking time to explain, honestly, the good and bad aspects of managing illness should nowadays be an essential part of every consultation between the patient and their doctor.

Everybody, including patients and their relatives, wants to know more about their health. *The Good Gut Guide* deals with intestinal diseases. Although this may at first seem to be a small part of the totality of medicine, intestinal diseases and problems are in fact very common. For example, Irritable Bowel Syndrome is one of the most frequent reasons for seeing a GP. While the condition is not life-threateningly serious, it accounts for a huge amount of suffering and has economic consequences because of time taken off work. Other intestinal diseases also have a great impact on individuals and society: infections, inflammatory bowel diseases such as ulcerative colitis and Crohn's disease, and cancers are all disabling – whether temporarily or more chronically – to millions of people.

Inflammatory bowel diseases affect young people. In some cases they can be very severe but in most, medical and surgical treatment can keep them under control, allowing the patient to lead a normal life. Bowel cancer is the second most common malignancy in our society, yet if diagnosed early it is curable. Polyps can give us early warning. These are tumours in the benign stage, and if removed, there is every chance that their evolution into cancer can be avoided. Indeed, cancer prevention by appropriate screening, increasingly through genetic indicators, offers a real opportunity for doctors to improve the results of cancer treatment.

Anal problems are extremely common. Although not serious, piles, abscesses and ulcers such as fissures can make life miserable for millions of sufferers. Incontinence may make life impossible, confining sufferers to staying at home near the toilet, too fearful to venture out to the shops let alone to social occasions such as parties or family gatherings. The good news is that these diseases are almost always treated successfully.

The Good Gut Guide is an impressive creation. It covers a vast field and includes just about every area that can be related to the intestine. It is accurate, well informed, practical and readable. It gives the medical facts in an authoritative and balanced manner and, at the same time, offers vital advice on the holistic aspects – such as diet and lifestyle – that are not usually available in normal medical books.

It will help patients and anyone else who wants to learn more about intestinal problems and improve their gut health.

PROFESSOR JOHN NICHOLLS

How I Came to Write This Book

When I first started suffering with proctitis in 1987, I was told it was a mild and localized form of ulcerative colitis, which was very unlikely to become serious or ever result in major surgery. Unfortunately, I was one of the unlucky few and 11 years later my entire large bowel was removed during a complex and lengthy operation.

It was very painful but, at the age of 34, I was more concerned about the prospect of wearing a 'bag' for the rest of my life. I mistakenly believed I'd have to wear baggy clothes and would never be able to enjoy scuba diving, swimming, or even lying on a beach again. However, I was given an 'internal pouch' instead. This involved reconfiguring my intestines to make part of my small bowel into a reservoir for digestive waste, meaning that I could continue to 'go to the bathroom' almost as normal. I thought it was great (despite a few practical limitations and the odd bout of 'pouchitis') – not only did it enable me to live without self-consciousness, I was finally free of my UC. I was bursting with energy and enthusiasm.

Having spent the better part of 10 years explaining my illness to people, I was amazed at how taboo the subject of bowels was. We seemed to be at the same stage of ignorance and silence that breast cancer sufferers were 30 or 40 years previously – when women were too ashamed to go to their doctor with a breast lump and when they, quite literally, died because of their embarrassment. But look at how all that has changed – with massive health and charity campaigns raising public awareness of this terrible illness.

I wanted to see the same revolution for sufferers of bowel diseases. So, just days after leaving hospital, I made an impulsive call to the *Daily Mail*'s Good Health Editor at the time, Rory Clements. Despite having never written for publication before, I offered to write him an article on my experience. Amazingly, he took up my offer and the full-page feature was duly published in March 1998. It marked the start of my efforts to take the taboo out of bowel illnesses.

So why write this book now? For the same reasons I made that phone call. Statistically, you are more likely to be killed by a donkey than *not* suffer with some gut-related problem at some time during your life. Many gut problems – including bowel cancers – are more easily and more successfully treated when they're picked up early. Taboos often prevent people from addressing problems until they are just too big and too serious to ignore, by which time it may be too late. Talk destroys taboos. Information saves lives.

I hope this book will help us to destroy the taboo, and enjoy good gut health.

Introduction

When I was 25 years old I experienced a disturbing symptom – bleeding from my bottom. Because I was then pregnant, I put it down to simple haemorrhoids and thought nothing more of it.

I never suspected that this was the beginning of a decade's worth of increasingly serious illness that I would face virtually alone, unaided and only vaguely informed. It wasn't the doctors' fault – they told me what, medically, I needed to know. And there were support groups, although I tended to notice only the people who suffered far worse than I did. Because of this, I shied away from associating with them – as if the seriousness of their illnesses might somehow be contagious.

Things that go wrong with your guts cause great embarrassment and this in turn makes them frightening. You don't automatically know who to talk to or what words to use, and when you do seek medical help the resulting procedures can be embarrassing as well as uncomfortable.

For some reason bowel and intestinal disorders have always been viewed as older people's afflictions, despite the fact that *most* cases of ulcerative colitis (UC), Crohn's disease and IBS start during a person's mid-twenties (or younger) – when many people are single, embarking on relationships, starting families or juggling demanding careers and busy social lives. I'm not sure why this false image has so stubbornly persisted, although I believe it is slowly changing.

As a health writer, I am regularly bombarded by information about new treatments – not just from orthodox medicine, but also from the herbal, dietary and complementary sides. My personal view is that the key to a 'golden cure' is not the preserve of any one of these camps. The answer to bowel illnesses is probably (and quite unsatisfactorily for those of us who like things neat and tidy) a complicated mixture of several elements, the proportions and exact ingredients of which we simply cannot isolate today. It's up to us to look carefully at every possibility, to try whatever we feel may be right for us, and work toward the best possible outcome – good gut health.

And that's why I've written this book – to provide the appropriate information so that the reader can play an active role in achieving good gut health. It isn't a book that features only a couple of gut problems in great detail. Neither is it a medical encyclopaedia that covers a whole raft of illnesses on a basic level. It is a user-friendly book for anyone who has ever experienced gut problems – and one that discusses them in a way that people understand.

This book looks at all types of intestinal symptoms – like diarrhoea, wind, constipation, nausea, abdominal pain and more – and offers practical solutions for dealing with them. Not just medical solutions, but self-help – including dietary and lifestyle tips, herbal help and a whole range of complementary therapies, from flower remedies to Ayurveda (an ancient Indian system of medicine). This approach is vital. People today are more proactive in choosing their healthcare than ever before and it is important to me that this book strongly reflects the diverse range of options now available.

Having looked at symptoms, the book then homes in on the diseases that are the key culprits of gut trouble and explains, simply but in detail, what these diseases are, what causes them, who they typically affect, what the risk factors are, how to prevent them and what medical treatments are available. Again, I have included practical advice for the patient in terms of self-help, dietary management, alternative treatments and prevention.

Lastly, the book focuses on the person behind the illness. It looks at the effect that chronic or embarrassing illnesses can have on our daily lives, our personalities and our relationships. It offers advice on the practicalities of living a normal life and coping with depression, hospitals, illness and surgery. There is also a large resource section at the back of the book for anyone who wants access to support groups, medical agencies and further information.

having trouble with

your guts?

———

What it means and what
you can do about it

Anything unusual that happens to our guts – like rampant diarrhoea or sudden bleeding – is disturbing. However, such occurrences are not the only reason we visit our doctor with a gut-related problem. Some common conditions like constipation are often mild, but they may gradually worsen until we become concerned enough to seek medical advice. You can just as easily need to see your doctor for a chronic problem as an acute one.

There are hundreds of medical problems – serious as well as minor ones – that cause 'gut-related' symptoms such as diarrhoea, constipation or mild stomach pains. This makes symptoms tricky to assess. How do we *know* when they are serious enough to warrant medical advice? Very few people get a thrill from visiting their doctor to be told that they are making a fuss but, on the other hand, what would happen if we ignored something serious?

Most digestive problems, whether serious or commonplace, don't present just one symptom. Usually we notice a couple, perhaps more. Here's an example: George notices that he's constipated, and occasionally sees flecks of bright red blood on the toilet paper; Sally feels a lot of discomfort when she goes to the toilet, especially when she is straining, and is also irritated by anal itching. George and Sally each have piles. They have the same condition, but they have differing symptoms. George's main problems are constipation and bleeding, Sally's are discomfort and itching. This is another reason why it is sometimes difficult to tell what is causing a particular health problem.

Analysing your symptoms in an almost detached way is part of the answer. For this reason, Section 1 focuses on the common symptoms like diarrhoea, constipation, bleeding, and wind and bloating. Very few of us wake up and think, 'I think I've got inflammatory bowel disease.' More likely we'll say, 'This diarrhoea is getting me down, I wonder what's causing it and how I can stop it.' This section explains what can cause these symptoms and offers a variety of practical ways we can help relieve them.

Section 1 also discusses how we can get the best from our doctors – by knowing what to ask, how to ask and what to expect from medical consultations, and describes the major tests that are used by doctors to explore and identify gut problems.

CHAPTER 1

A Quick Anatomy Lesson

First, let's go back to the classroom. It is easier to understand why things go wrong – and how we are affected – if we know a little about the anatomy of the gut.

The digestive system starts at our mouth and ends up at the other end – the anus. When people talk about 'guts' they can mean pretty much anything, from the throat to the stomach to the intestines, although generally, most people think of the stomach and the small and large intestines when they say 'gut'. Vagueness may be okay when we're chatting with friends, but there's little room for it in the doctor's office. Being specific helps our doctors understand what we're talking about. We might think we're being fairly exact when we say 'abdominal', but a doctor could easily wonder whether we mean the stomach, the small intestines or the large bowel (colon and rectum). And should he ask which it is, it helps to know what he's talking about.

A few minutes spent looking at the drawing overleaf should help. This shows the whole digestive system, its various parts and their medical names. The other diagrams provide a little more detail about the lining of the intestines. There are different layers, each of which performs different functions. The whole of the digestive system is hugely vascular (that is, rich in blood vessels). A staggering quantity of blood passes through it – some 40 per cent of our blood supply is diverted through the digestive system after a meal, so that the blood can absorb the goodness our food delivers to our bodies. That's why it isn't a good idea to embark on strenuous exercise soon after eating – it puts too many demands on our body systems.

3

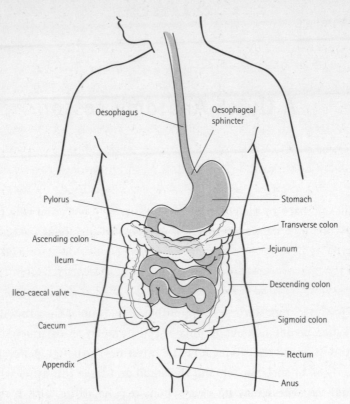

Oesophagus

Oesophageal sphincter

Pylorus

Stomach

Transverse colon

Ascending colon

Jejunum

Ileum

Ileo-caecal valve

Descending colon

Caecum

Sigmoid colon

Rectum

Appendix

Anus

The Mouth to the Oesophagus

The mouth is the first organ of digestion. Teeth chew our food, physically breaking it down, and the inside of our mouth contains glands that produce saliva – not only when we eat food but also when we're just thinking about it. Saliva is important. This liquid, which is neutral to slightly acidic, not only starts the chemical process of digestion, but it lubricates each mouthful, helping us to swallow properly. We produce about 1.7 litres (about 60fl oz) of saliva every day. One of the main enzymes contained in saliva is called amylase, which starts breaking starch down into more basic sugars. When we swallow, food enters the first 'tube' – the oesophagus, which is about 25cm (10in) long. The oesophagus doesn't do anything to digest food. Waves of muscle contraction (called peristalsis) help push the food down the oesophagus. These muscular contractions are so strong that you can drink a glass of water while standing on your head.

The Stomach

Food enters the stomach through a ring of muscle (sphincter) that prevents the stomach contents from travelling back up the oesophagus – the one normal exception to this is during vomiting. The stomach is so stretchy that it can hold up to 2 litres (about 70fl oz) of fluid. While food is in the stomach it is subjected to both physical and chemical action. Stomach acids – mostly hydrochloric acid (one of the strongest acids known to man) – reduce the stomach contents to a porridge-like consistency, while the stomach also mechanically 'churns' the food during the four hours or so that food stays there. Because the stomach contents are very acidic, we get 'burning' sensations when we vomit, have indigestion or gastric reflux, as the contents bubble back up into the oesophagus. After a while, the sphincter muscle (called the pylorus) that holds the lower end of the stomach closed starts to relax, allowing the partly-digested food to trickle out into the first portion of the small intestine.

The Small Intestine

As food is squirted through the pylorus, it enters the first part of the small intestine, the duodenum. Here, more digestive chemicals are introduced, further breaking down the food. Bile, for example, an alkaline substance that is made in the liver, is pumped out by the gall bladder when needed. Bile acts as a detergent and emulsifying agent, breaking fats down into small droplets. Pancreatic enzymes break down carbohydrates and proteins: amylase acts on carbohydrates and trypsin and chymotrypsin help digest proteins. Fats are also further broken down by lipase, another pancreatic enzyme.

The next section of the small intestine, the 3 metre (10ft) long jejunum, is where most of the nutrients released from food start to be absorbed. The walls of the jejunum are completely covered with tiny finger-like projections called villi. Millions of these millimetre-high folds line the intestinal walls, their purpose being to massively increase the surface area to make absorption of nutrients into the bloodstream effective (see figure overleaf). If the small intestines didn't have villi, they would need to be about 2 miles long to do the same job – in fact, they are only about 6 metres (20ft) long. After

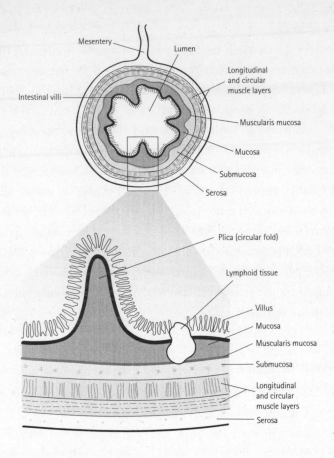

the jejunum comes another 3 metre (10ft) long section of small bowel commonly known as the ileum. Although there are still many villi here, there are fewer than in the jejunum. The ileum continues to absorb nutrients into the bloodstream, but the focus here is more on water and salts; as food progresses through the small bowel, the consistency of it becomes thicker and more 'sludgy'. In the very last part of the ileum, vitamin B12 is absorbed.

The Large Intestine – the Colon, Rectum and Anus

Once food has travelled through the small intestine, most of the essential nourishment has already been absorbed. What enters the colon is watery slurry. It passes through the ileo-caecal valve into a stretchy section of the colon called the caecum. The appendix hangs down from the caecum and is a relic, doctors believe, from when the human diet was far higher in plant matter than it is today. The appendix may have contained special bacterial agents that digest cellulose – much like grass-eating animals have. In the colon, water is reabsorbed from the watery slurry, making the waste more solid. What have now become faeces ('poo') slowly travel along the last portion of the colon until they reach the rectum, where they are expelled through the anus.

Bacteria flourish in huge numbers in the colon. Even though they are present in the stomach and the small intestines, there is generally too much activity (and acidity) in these areas for them to thrive. But in the colon, the waste passes through much more slowly and the environment becomes increasingly alkaline, allowing bacteria to multiply in vast numbers. However, these bacteria serve a useful purpose – not only do they help break down much of the remaining undigested material, but they also reduce the wind that is generated as waste slowly passes through the colon. There are exchanges of various hormones as well – for example, excess oestrogen in the blood is passed through the walls of the colon, and, if the diet is high in fibre, it binds to this fibre and can then be excreted. Otherwise, it would be reabsorbed back into the blood. Scientists now realize that too much of certain oestrogens in the body can be a contributory factor in the development of many 'hormonal' cancers – like breast cancer, ovarian and cervical cancers, even prostate and testicular cancers in men. Minerals can also be reabsorbed into the body here.

Food travels slowly through the colon – the average journey time is 12–48 hours to get through this $1^1/2$–2 metre (5–6ft) long tube. The colon walls secrete mucus to lubricate the waste matter and help it move along smoothly. In fact, mucus-secretion happens all the way along the gut – coming from a thin layer of cells called the mucous membrane. This membrane also protects the gut wall against bacteria and the acidity of the digestive enzymes, and helps ensure that it is our food and not our gut that gets digested when we eat. The rectum is about 15cm (6in) long and lies between the colon and the anal canal. It acts as a reservoir for the faeces. When it becomes full, nerve endings trigger strong muscular contractions that make us want to empty our bowels. This happens when the anal sphincter muscles open, allowing the waste to be expelled.

CHAPTER 2

Common Symptoms

Now we've had a quick glance at the anatomy of the digestive system, it is time to look at the symptoms that can indicate a gut problem.

This book *cannot* give you a definitive diagnosis – only your doctor can – but it can point you in the right direction. The self-help sections for each symptom offer practical advice on what *you* can do to help alleviate your problem.

Please note that you should **always seek urgent medical help** if any of the following occur:

- Severe abdominal pain.
- Acute diarrhoea and vomiting lasting more than 24 hours in the case of adults or 4–6 hours for infants, the elderly and anyone with a pre-existing medical condition.
- Bleeding from the back passage.
- Vomiting blood.

Constipation

'Tell someone you're constipated and sometimes they judge your personality more than your body. Phrases like "anally retentive" and "tight-arse" seem to spring into some people's minds. I can almost see some people thinking it, although perhaps I'm over-sensitive. But I'm not tight-arsed, I'm not hung-up or repressed, and I'm not scared of "letting go". I do, however, have a problem with constipation!'

Adrian, 46, who regularly suffers from constipation

Constipation is not a disease, but simply a sign that our intestines are having trouble getting rid of compacted waste in our bowels. The majority of cases of constipation are caused by simple problems like dehydration, changes in routine (like travelling), ignoring the body's 'urges' to go and even things like iron supplements and certain common medicines (like those containing codeine). Constipation can also happen during pregnancy, and is often associated with piles, or encopresis (a childhood problem). An underactive thyroid may also cause constipation, as can IBS and proctitis. Diverticular disease can be caused by chronic constipation. More serious, but also more rare, causes of constipation include intestinal obstruction, botulism poisoning, typhoid and paratyphoid, and bowel cancer.

Constipation is one of the most common afflictions of modern, westernized society – only 40 per cent of men and 33 per cent of women open their bowels regularly once a day and, according to surveys, over $4^1/2$ million Americans say they are constipated most or all of the time. Constipation is far less common in developing cultures where the diet is predominantly vegetarian. Highly refined and low-fibre products, fast foods and too many fatty or sugary foods are the main culprits of this problem.

There is also a mental element to constipation; a Gallup survey recently revealed that more than half of us are put off by the idea of using public toilets when out shopping and one in four of us feel the same hesitation over using toilets in restaurants or bars. The main reason for this is being unsure of the hygiene of public toilets – but there's more to it than cleanliness. Millions of holidaymakers suffer with constipation. It's a common phenomenon that has a lot to do with the disruption of routines and with being in unfamiliar circumstances. Stress may also play a part.

How Do You Know If You're Constipated?

Bowel habits are an individual thing. Some people go twice a day, while others may go only every other day. Generally, anything between three times a day and three times a week is considered 'normal', although there are perfectly healthy people whose toilet habits fall outside even this broad range. 'Normal' is what is normal for *you* and not anyone else. Judge it by your own daily habits. Another sign of constipation is when you pass stools that are small and hard – so-called 'rabbit pellets'.

What Helps Relieve Constipation?

Fibrous food adds bulk without calories – a bonus for anyone trying to lose weight – and also helps our intestines move digestive waste through (and out of) our bodies. Exercise, drinking plenty of water and increasing your fibre intake are often all that is needed to help remedy constipation. In developed countries people use laxatives far more often than necessary; laxatives can potentially aggravate things because they don't address the root cause of constipation and may encourage the guts to become inactive without them. (Stimulant laxatives work by speeding up the muscular movements of our gut, forcing our waste food to be eliminated much more quickly than normal.) The same goes for enemas: according to the National Digestive Diseases Information Clearinghouse, the regular use of enemas 'can impair the natural muscle action of the intestines, leaving them unable to function normally'.

Self-Help for Constipation

- **Fluids:** Drink more water – aim for an intake of at least 2 litres (4 pints) of water daily. And watch your intake of tea and coffee as they may make constipation worse.
- **Fibre:** Eating high-fibre foods as part of your everyday diet, is an easy way of alleviating chronic constipation (although some people suffering from IBS may find that fibre can aggravate their symptoms). However, be careful to increase your fibre intake slowly (especially with beans and pulses) – a rapid change can result in a marked increase in wind and abdominal discomfort, although this normally lessens as your guts get used to the change in diet. The recommended amount of fibre in the diet is about 20–35 grams a day. Try the following suggestions:
  - Choose wholemeal or added-fibre bread and pasta, brown rice and unrefined flour.
  - Eat more fruit and vegetables.
  - Bran can be added to the diet, especially cereals.
  - Flaxseed is a good source of soluble and insoluble fibre (3 grams per tablespoon, which is a lot), as well as contributing omega-3 fatty acids. Sprinkle it over salads and cereals or yoghurt to give a nutty taste. You can also substitute ground flaxseed for flour (in small quantities).

- Dried apricots, desiccated coconut, dried peaches and toasted almonds are all very high in fibre and are convenient snacks.
- **Eat regular meals:** The digestive system responds best when we eat little and often. Also try to have your main meal of the day at lunchtime to give it time to digest properly during the afternoon.
- **Exercise:** A healthy, exercised body always functions more efficiently than an underactive one, and the bowels respond just as happily to exercise as our heart and cardiovascular system does. Even if it's a brisk 30-minute walk three times a week, or a gentle swim, try and work exercise into your routine.
- **Don't ignore urges:** Try your best not to ignore the call of nature when you feel it. It's difficult if you're out, or cannot find a clean toilet, or are a shift worker whose body clock is all over the place, but do persevere all the same.
- **Establish helpful routines:** The bowels love routine. If sitting on the loo with your daily newspaper for a few minutes every morning helps you get a regular routine going, then do it.
- **Avoid laxatives:** Most people need to resort to laxatives every once in a while, but where possible they should be avoided – especially stimulant laxatives. Overuse of laxatives can lead to dependency, which is not healthy for the bowels and can cause unwelcome changes in the bowel if used for many years.
- **Herbal help:** Laxatives – herbal or otherwise – are not a long-term solution to constipation but there are several herbs with mild purgative properties that can be used occasionally. Senna is the best known, but there are several others, including cascara, frangula, and yellow dock. They all contain special plant chemicals called anthraquinone glycosides, which have a laxative effect. Other herbs known for their ability to help relieve constipation include aloes, dandelion, liquorice, and rhubarb root. Ispaghula husk is an excellent natural bulking agent, which helps the body move waste food through the large intestine more easily. It should always be taken with *lots* of water.
- **Aromatherapy:** Marjoram, rosemary and fennel oil may help; put a few drops into a base oil and gently rub onto the abdomen.
- **Homeopathy:** There are several homeopathic remedies for various types of occasional constipation. These include lycopodeum, nux vomica, sepia, silicea, bryonia and alumina.

■ **Further Information:**
National Digestive Diseases Information Clearinghouse,
www.niddk.nih.gov/health/digest/pubs/const/const.htm and
www.niddk.nih.gov/health/digest/pubs/whyconst/whyconst.htm
For constipation in children, see Digestive Disorders Foundation,
www.digestivedisorders.org.uk/Leaflets/adconsNEW.html

Laxatives – What Are They?

Laxatives are substances that encourage the bowels to open. They are
extraordinarily popular – nearly $1 billion is spent on laxatives each year in
the US. There are several types:

■ **Bulking agents** are concentrated fibre preparations that include bran,
ispaghula husk, methylcellulose and sterculia. Brand names to look for
include Fybogel and Isogel (UK), Metamucil and Citrucel (US). All bulking
agents should be taken with plenty of water, as this helps them to swell
and form their bulk, which in turn helps move waste effectively through
the large intestine.

■ **Stimulant laxatives** encourage bowel movements by stimulating the nerve
endings in the bowel walls to make the muscles contract. This speeding up
of bowel muscles encourages waste to pass through more quickly. In doing
so, less water is reabsorbed back through the bowel walls into the body,
the stools retain more moisture, are less dense and compacted, and
therefore easier to pass. Stimulant laxatives can cause diarrhoea if taken
too often or in overdose and dependency can develop with overuse. They
should not be used for longer than a week at a time and never given to
children without a doctor's specific advice. Brands include Dulco-Lax and
Senokot (both UK and US).

■ **Lubricants and stool softeners** such as liquid paraffin, mineral oil and
glycerine suppositories can be given to help soften hard, impacted faeces.
They are most often used when haemorrhoids or anal fissures cause severe
pain on straining.

■ **Osmotic laxatives** such as Epsom salts are used to attract more water into
the bowel, which then softens hard stools. They can cause chemical
imbalances in the blood and aren't generally recommended for long-term

use. Lactulose and sorbitol sugars also act as osmotic agents and are often used as an alternative to bulking agents in the long-term treatment of chronic constipation. Lactulose should never be used by anyone with lactose intolerance or milk allergy.

Diarrhoea

'Everyone knows it – first, you get a gripey feeling deep in your belly, then you know you've got just a few seconds or less to get yourself into the nearest loo. It's something that babies in nappies wouldn't care about, but as an adult it becomes a real social problem. If it's an acute case of food poisoning or holiday tummy it's bad enough, but to have it constantly is a different ball-game altogether. It changes your life completely. You can't go anywhere or do anything without military planning and knowing where every toilet is located. You become really good at inventing excuses and avoiding intimate situations. I've even had to resort to carrying spare underwear and wet wipes because of the odd disaster.'

Graham, 22, who suffers from severe, urgent diarrhoea caused by ulcerative colitis

Diarrhoea is defined as 'frequent passing of abnormally loose or watery faeces', and most of us easily know when we're suffering from it! The urge to get to the bathroom quickly is normally a main feature and occasionally the first time we know we've got diarrhoea is when we're 'caught short' or break 'wet' wind. Faecal incontinence (the medical term for being caught short) is more common than you might think, affecting one in 20 of us at some time or another.

Diarrhoea is often, though not always, accompanied by stomach cramps and, if it is caused by food poisoning, food intolerance or a flu-like illness, you may feel sick and throw up as well. Diarrhoea can be acute, starting suddenly and lasting only for a short period of time, or chronic and linger for weeks, months or years.

What Causes Diarrhoea?

The guts are very susceptible to developing diarrhoea – excess caffeine, vigorous exercise, excess fibre, excess alcohol, stress, antibiotics and even medicines and supplements (like iron, for example) can all cause it. Food intolerance and coeliac disease can also induce diarrhoea and in children it may be associated with a condition called encopresis. An overactive thyroid can cause diarrhoea, but so can viral gastroenteritis, parasitic infections, food poisoning, malabsorption, IBS, polyps and proctitis. While diarrhoea is far more likely to be caused by a minor problem, it can occasionally indicate more serious problems like ulcerative colitis, Crohn's disease, diverticulitis, appendicitis, TSS, typhoid or paratyphoid, cholera and bowel cancer.

How Should I Treat Diarrhoea?

The first and most important thing is not to become dehydrated. This is especially important for babies, young children and the elderly, who dehydrate far more quickly than adults. Dehydration has all sorts of serious knock-on effects as it upsets the finely tuned balance of body salts and essential nutrients; in serious cases it can even lead to brain damage and death. An infant or child with diarrhoea is soon at significant risk of dehydration, so always take action quickly and seek medical help if it persists for more than 6 hours. Babies cannot tell you how they feel, but in infants under 18 months old, the fontanelle (the space between the growing skull bones that can be felt on the top of a baby's head) may look sunken. In both babies and adults the urine will be a dark yellow colour and hardly any will be produced at all. Other symptoms include having a dry mouth and lips, and lethargy.

When to Seek Help

An attack of diarrhoea can pass very quickly, but if it is severe, prolonged or accompanied by bleeding seek medical advice urgently. In children and the elderly, diarrhoea can rapidly become very serious, if not life threatening, and help should be sought quickly.

Self-Help for Diarrhoea

■ Fluids: If you have diarrhoea *and* vomiting, it may not be a good idea to drink much for a while, until your stomach can handle a few sips of water. Otherwise, if you're unaffected by sickness, drink plenty of fluids – bottled water and soft drinks. If you're abroad and think you may have 'traveller's diarrhoea', avoid all tap water and any drinks containing ice cubes, as these may have been made from tap water.

- **Balance your electrolytes:** Rehydration salts like Dioralyte and Rehidrat are widely available at pharmacies and most supermarkets or grocery stores. These are important as they help restore vital salts like sodium (common salt) and potassium, which are easily lost with diarrhoea. In emergencies, you can easily make your own using basic kitchen ingredients – put a generous pinch of salt and one teaspoon of sugar into 250ml (8fl oz) of cooled boiled water, bottled water or fruit juice.

- **Anti-diarrhoeal medicines:** These are also widely available in stores, pharmacies and airports – look for the drug name 'loperamide' or brands like Arret, Diocalm Ultra, Enterocalm and Imodium. Another useful drug is diphenoxylate (Lomotil). These medicines are especially useful if you're travelling and can't rely on finding a toilet when you want. However, avoid anti-diarrhoeal medicines if you have severe stomach pains or are bleeding – instead, seek medical advice urgently.

- **Lower the fibre:** Sometimes too much fibre can cause diarrhoea. Children and weaning infants are particularly prone as their digestive systems are not yet used to large quantities of fibrous foods.

- **Lower the fat:** Highly fatty foods can aggravate diarrhoea.

- **Cut down on food:** Your stomach doesn't want a rich or a heavy meal while you've got diarrhoea. Cut down on dairy products and fatty, fried and spicy foods, and stick to light meals and bland foods – crackers, wafers, breadsticks, bananas, soups and broths. Carrot juice may be helpful.

- **Take care with food and personal hygiene:** Many cases of diarrhoea are caused by food poisoning and although it can be serious enough to kill, in most instances food poisoning only results in nausea and/or diarrhoea. Around 100,000 cases of food poisoning are reported in England and Wales every year, although microbiologist Professor Glenn Gibson at Reading University estimates the real figure is up to 20 times higher, because so many cases are mild and therefore go unreported.

- **Check your medicines:** Diarrhoea can be a side effect of many medicines. Check with your pharmacist or doctor that your current medication isn't causing your diarrhoea, especially if it started around the same time that you began taking the drug.

- **Antibiotics:** Occasionally, your doctor may prescribe a course of antibiotics to treat diarrhoea. Antibiotics should never be taken in order to *prevent* diarrhoea. Bear in mind that some types of antibiotic may *cause* mild diarrhoea.

- **Herbal medicines:** Many herbs possess anti-diarrhoeal properties; some, like German chamomile and thyme, are especially useful for treating infant diarrhoea. Chamomile can also be used to help relieve nervous diarrhoea, while garden burnet has traditionally been used to treat acute diarrhoea attacks. Raspberry leaf may also help. Peppermint oil, which acts as an anti-spasmodic agent, can help reduce the stomach cramps that sometimes accompany diarrhoea.

- **Supplements:** Taking live bacteria (probiotics) after an attack of diarrhoea has passed will help repopulate your gut with 'friendly' bacteria. They come in the form of yoghurts, drinks and tablets or capsules. They are especially useful if they are 'enteric-coated' – that is, protected by a chemical coating so that strong stomach acids cannot kill them. It means that more of the bacteria reach the small and large intestines alive. Check product labels: Lactobacilli (*L. acidophilus*) and Bifidobacteria (*B. longum and B. bifidum*) are good bacterial strains.

- **Chinese herbal medicine:** Skullcap root can be useful for treating acute diarrhoea; so can dandelion root and golden thread.

- **Further information:** Digestive Disorders Foundation, www.digestivedisorders.org.uk/Leaflets/diarrhoeNEW.html

Nausea

'Feeling sick' is a symptom of a myriad of illnesses, many of which are directly linked to the digestive system. Food intolerance is commonly associated with nausea. Other diet-related conditions like coeliac disease and food poisoning cause nausea and vomiting, as can gastritis, viral gastroenteritis, peptic ulcers, IBS and most parasitic infections. More serious conditions that can contribute to feelings of nausea include Crohn's disease, diverticulitis, appendicitis, peritonitis, Toxic Shock Syndrome (TSS), intussusception (a condition affecting infants), botulism and cholera.

However, not all cases of nausea can be attributed to problems of the digestive system. Many common occurrences, like hangovers or migraines, induce nausea. It can also be caused by emotional states like nervousness, fright and excitement, and by psychological disturbances like bulimia. Nausea, especially in the morning, is a common symptom of early pregnancy.

Note: If you suspect you may be pregnant, have this confirmed as soon as possible. Pregnant women must be careful about what they eat, drink and take in the way of medication. Even everyday drugs that are available without prescription may be harmful to a baby, as are smoking and alcohol. Many herbal preparations are advised against during pregnancy, due to lack of information about their possible side effects. Always consult your doctor before taking ANY health preparations if you are, or might be, pregnant.

When to Seek Help

If you experience severe abdominal pain with your nausea, or bloodstained vomit, seek urgent medical advice.

Self-Help for Nausea

- **Sip cold water:** If you have mild nausea, taking small sips of very cold water (or sucking ice cubes) can help. Don't take large gulps, because too much liquid on a queasy stomach may make you sick.
- **Deep breathing:** If there is an element of stress or anxiety in your nausea, take a series of slow, deep breaths in through the nose and out through the mouth.
- **Take a short walk in fresh air:** A gentle walk in fresh air can sometimes help relieve nausea, especially if you are stuck in a stuffy room, are overheated, or are in an air-conditioned office. A short walk also improves the circulation.
- **Aromatherapy:** Peppermint oil is useful if nausea troubles you – aromatherapy oils can be used in gentle massage, or as a relieving fragrance.
- **Herbal relief:** Peppermint and chamomile teas can quell nausea. Ginger is also known for its anti-nausea properties (especially good for travel sickness and pregnancy sickness) – try ginger tea or eating small pieces of crystallized ginger. Scientists believe that ginger neutralizes gut toxins and acids and slows down the feedback between the nerves of the stomach and the part of the brain that controls nausea.

- **Homeopathy:** Sepia (a derivative of cuttlefish) is often used to ease nausea, as are nux vomica and arsenicum (if nausea is accompanied by diarrhoea).
- **Flower remedies:** Rescue Remedy (available from most health food stores) is calming and can be useful when vomiting causes distress or is associated with worry or panic.
- **Vitamins:** Vitamin B6 can help alleviate morning sickness, but check with your doctor first that it is safe for you to take. If you're already taking multi-vitamins, make sure you're not doubling-up.
- **Further Information:**
  Altruis Biomedical Network, www.gastrointestinal.net/

Bleeding

'When it first happened, I was 28 and only three months' pregnant with my first child, so to sit on the loo and discover I was bleeding gave me an enormous fright. At first I thought I was having a miscarriage – my heart stopped beating and I was shaking. After a minute or so, I realized it wasn't because of the baby, but was coming from behind. I was relieved, of course, that it wasn't a miscarriage, but still shocked to see blood, even when I guessed it was probably just something simple like haemorrhoids.

I have since experienced a lot of bleeding, as I've had problems with haemorrhoids through all four of my pregnancies. And you know what? It still unnerves me, because even though I know it won't kill me, I also know it's not "normal" '.

Gill, 42, a mother-of-four, who has been troubled by haemorrhoids for many years

How Can You Tell if You're Bleeding?

The answer may seem obvious – bright red blood passing out of your bowel. You'd be a fool not to notice, right? Well, not necessarily. People are often in a hurry, preoccupied or distracted, and some of us are more likely to make a visual inspection of our bowel movements than others. It's human nature – we all have different levels (and areas) of curiosity. If bleeding comes from high up in the digestive system, it may not look bright red at all, but may be black and tarry – we may not even recognize it as blood. Similarly, women having a period may easily confuse blood that actually comes from their bowels with menstrual flow. Lastly, blood may occasionally be present even though we don't see it at all – this is called 'occult', or hidden, bleeding and can be tested for by doctors.

Because doctors take bleeding seriously, they will normally ask several questions about it, so it's a good idea to think about when and how your bleeding shows itself. What colour is it? Is it bright red or dark, even black? Is it mixed in with your stools, or does it appear as a streak on the toilet paper? Does it only happen during a bowel movement, or at other times as well? Have you noticed any other symptoms like diarrhoea, pain, tiredness or itching?

What is Bleeding a Sign Of?

Bleeding, although it may be alarming, doesn't necessarily mean that there is a serious problem. It is actually a fairly common complaint, affecting over 15 per cent of us at some point or other in our lives.

Bleeding happens for many reasons. The delicate lining of our stomach and intestines is highly vascular – this means that millions of small blood vessels are extremely close to the surface in order for our blood to absorb the nutrients we need as food progresses through the gut. Anything that upsets this lining is likely to cause bleeding. *Helicobacter pylori*, the bacterium that is now known to cause the majority of stomach and duodenal ulcers, irritates the gut lining and makes it bleed. (Even an excess of alcohol can irritate the delicate lining and cause tiny blood vessels to rupture, spilling blood into the digestive tract.) Simply treated problems like haemorrhoids are the most common cause of bleeding, although proctitis, polyps, anal fistulas, anal fissures and rectal prolapses can also cause it. The most serious causes of bleeding from the back passage include intussusception (in children), diverticulitis, ulcerative colitis, Crohn's disease, bowel cancer and anal cancer.

When to Seek Help

A doctor must always check bleeding. However, it is usually caused by a minor problem, so don't let any signs of bleeding send you into an uncontrolled panic.

Self-Help for Bleeding

- **Check your diet:** Certain foods can make you think you're bleeding when you're not. Beetroot, for instance, can make the stools look red. So can blueberries and other highly-coloured foodstuffs. Iron can make stools look black.
- **Identify the source:** This isn't always easy to do, but there are clues. Bright red blood from the anus is likely to be coming from nearby – the lower colon, rectum or anus. Darker blood will be from higher up. Black, tarry-like substances generally indicate bleeding from the stomach or small intestine.
- **When does it happen?** Do you notice bleeding all the time or only when you pass a stool? Identifying the timing of bleeding can give your doctor good clues as to the cause.
- **Think about other symptoms:** Is your bleeding accompanied by diarrhoea or constipation? Do you have any abdominal pain? Is there any sharp or severe pain in your bottom? Do you feel nauseous or sick?
- **Look at your medicine chest:** Have you been taking any medicines recently – especially aspirin, non-steroidal anti-inflammatory drugs (NSAIDs, such as ibuprofen, naproxen) or other drugs? Some medicines can aggravate ulcers and cause them to bleed.
- **Rectal bleeding:** If you are bleeding because of haemorrhoids or a split in the skin around the anus, a dab of olive oil can encourage healing and reduce pain – so too can witch hazel, which also reduces the inflammation associated with piles.
- **Further Information:**
  National Digestive Diseases Information Clearinghouse,
  www.niddk.nih.gov/health/digest/pubs/bleeding/bleeding.htm

Mucus

Mucus is a slimy secretion that is constantly produced by virtually the entire gastrointestinal tract. Special cells are responsible for producing the mucus secretions, which coat the gastric and intestinal membranes. Mucus helps not only to protect the sensitive lining of the stomach and intestines against the strong acids that digest our food, but it also helps food slide more easily through our guts. The reason we don't normally see it is because the mucus becomes bound up with faecal waste matter, becoming invisible in the process.

What Can Mucus Be a Sign Of?

In itself, mucus is an innocent and harmless by-product of the digestive process. But there are occasions when we may notice it. If we've been unwell and not eating, it is possible that some mucus will be visible when we open our bowels, although it will still be mixed up with other body secretions, like bile from the gall bladder. People who have had their colon surgically 'disconnected' from their anus always notice that they start to discharge mucus from their tail end. It was ever thus, but once waste food matter is no longer being shunted through the anus, the one thing that *is* still being produced in that area – mucus – becomes very obvious.

Haemorrhoids are probably the most common cause of mucus discharge from the anus. Other causes of mucus include proctitis, polyps, anal fistulas, rectal prolapses, ulcerative colitis, bowel and anal cancer. Intussusception – a problem seen in young infants – causes red, jelly-like stools or bloodstained mucus. Even IBS can stimulate areas of the gut to produce more mucus. (It is interesting to note that IBS often used to be called 'mucous colitis'.)

Self-Help for Excess Mucus

- Have you been unwell? If you've not been eating, perhaps because of a stomach bug, you might notice more mucus. It will 'disappear' once your diet is back to normal.
- Are there any other symptoms? Look out for other symptoms – abdominal cramping, diarrhoea, urgency or frequency in going to the bathroom. Excess mucus can also indicate an infection.
- Avoid anal 'play': It may sound obvious, but if there's anything amiss with your tail end, it's best to leave it alone. That means avoiding anal intercourse or any other kind of love play that involves inserting foreign objects into the rectum.
- Herbal help: Both bayberry and witch hazel are purported to offer relief from 'mucous colitis' (IBS) and related conditions. Ask your herbalist for a suitable preparation, but only after you've identified the reason for your excess mucus.
- Homeopathy: Alumina may help if your mucus is accompanied by constipation. Argentum nitricum may help if you have wind, alternating

constipation and diarrhoea and mucus (symptoms typical in IBS sufferers, for example).

Abdominal Pain

How do you describe abdominal pain? There are lots of words because there are lots of different types of abdominal pain: there are dull aches, dragging sensations, sharp stabbing pains, intermittent ones – most of us have had 'tummy ache' at one time or another since childhood and we become pretty good at describing the various types. Of course, some tummy aches are minor – the results of eating too many chocolate eggs at Easter, for instance – but others can be agonizing pains that literally floor us. They often feel worse when we don't know what is causing them: fear is a highly aggravating factor in our perception of pain.

Pain in the abdomen is like pain in any other part of our bodies, warning us that something is not quite right. Our expectations of a pain-free life often lead us to view pain itself as the problem – we imagine that if we can get rid of the pain, the problem is automatically resolved. Not so. Pain is an alarm device that lets us know our bodies are not functioning properly. Pain should be listened to.

Fear, worry, stress and anxiety can subtly alter our perception of pain and can, in some cases, make us feel pain where, medically, there isn't any. It's what lies behind so-called 'psychosomatic' illnesses – diseases that our minds can trick us into believing we have. The mind is a very complex organ that scientists still do not understand and it can change our perception of pain in both negative and positive ways. One little girl I know quite happily had several dental fillings done with no anaesthetic, simply because she had overheard her father saying that he never used any anaesthetic when he visited the dentist. The motivating force – her father's approval – was enough to make her cope with the pain. When we are strongly motivated, we feel pain less intensely.

The fact that emotional states can affect our perception of pain makes it notoriously difficult to assess. And to compound this further, scientists have found that people have different pain thresholds, making one person's 'agony' another's 'discomfort'.

An Important Word about Pain and Pregnancy

It is quite common for abdominal pain to occur mid to late pregnancy
(especially if it's a first pregnancy), as the ligaments and muscles of the
abdomen stretch to accommodate the quickly growing baby. However, if you
experience any abdominal pain during any stage of pregnancy, always see your
doctor. **Self-diagnosis is not advisable during pregnancy and can be
dangerous.**

What Causes It?

Abdominal pain is probably the one symptom that has the widest range
of possible causes. These include period pains, excess alcohol, stress, overuse
of aspirin and food intolerance. Abdominal pain can also be caused by problems that aren't related to the gut – like the sexually-transmitted disease
chlamydia, or by ovarian cysts or ovarian cancer, or even by adhesions.
Abdominal pain is a common symptom of gut infections and infestations
such as viral gastroenteritis, parasitic infections, food poisoning,
gastritis, typhoid and paratyphoid. It can also be caused by inflammatory
conditions including proctitis, Crohn's disease, diverticulitis, appendicitis
and peritonitis. And various other problems may lead to abdominal pain of
varying degrees and locations – anal abscesses, hernias, peptic ulcers, malabsorption, IBS, bowel and gastric cancer, and intestinal obstruction.

Pain sensations are caused when pain receptors (special nerve endings
found throughout the body) are activated. They are usually triggered by
pressure on the nerve endings – for example, the sharp pressure of an injury
or the dull pressure of an increase in blood flow or fluid retention. The
receptors then send electrical impulses travelling along our nerves to
the brain, where they are interpreted as pain. Because the distribution of
pain receptors is highly uneven throughout the body, certain pains are felt
more distinctly than others. For example, there are probably more pain
receptors on the tongue alone than there are throughout the rest of the
digestive tract combined.

When to Seek Help

Any abdominal pain that is severe or lasts for longer than a couple of hours should be referred to a doctor, especially in children and infants, and urgently if there is also abdominal distension, the belly is rigid or swollen, if there is any bleeding or bloody vomit, or there is a fever.

Self-Help for Abdominal Pain

- **Identify the type of pain:** Some pains are crampy, others a dull ache. Some are constant, others intermittent. The more accurately you can describe the type and location of your pain, the easier it may be for your doctor to make an accurate diagnosis.
- **Women:** Make a note of where you are in your menstrual cycle – many abdominal pains are related to the reproductive organs rather than the digestive organs. Menstrual pain can be helped by holding a warm hot-water bottle on the abdomen, and by taking painkillers specifically designed to relieve menstrual cramps (for example, Feminax).
- **Diet:** If you have severe abdominal pain, do not eat anything, especially if you are vomiting. If your pains are crampy and intermittent, keep your diet very light and eat small snacks regularly, rather than one or two large meals through the day.
- **Relaxation techniques:** Scientific studies indicate that stress management techniques and relaxation skills (like hypnosis, repeating relaxing 'mantras', imagery to visualize pain relief, meditation and yoga) may all help reduce the perception of pain, particularly in chronic disorders like ulcerative colitis.
- **Herbal help:** Several herbs are stated to possess antispasmodic properties, which makes them useful if you suffer from colicky-type pain. They include asafoetida, cinnamon, ginger, lemon verbena, parsley, pennyroyal and valerian. Other herbs may help: calamus for intestinal colic and chaparral for bowel cramps.
- **Aromatherapy massage:** Chamomile and geranium essential oils, massaged into the abdomen, may help bring temporary relief.

Pain in the Back Passage

Gut problems can sometimes affect the rectum and anal areas – causing what we colloquially refer to as a 'pain in the butt'. Pain that affects the rectum and anus, however, is generally caused by problems specific to that area. These include haemorrhoids, proctitis, anal abscesses, anal fistulas and anal fissures. Pain in this area can also (occasionally) be caused by ulcerative colitis and Crohn's disease, and rarely by anal cancer.

The rectum and anus contain a lot more nerve endings than sections of the intestine that are deep inside our bodies. It is therefore much more likely that problems in this area will cause us to feel pain.

Self-Help for Pain in the Back Passage

- **Soreness due to diarrhoea:** Creams designed for nappy rash, like Sudocrem, can help. Make sure that your hygiene is scrupulous. Wash the area after every attack of diarrhoea (bidets are helpful), or if you're at work, carry a travel pack of moist toilet wipes with you. Gently pat the skin dry after washing, and apply cream.
- **Clothing:** Wear loose, cotton underwear to prevent chafing and overheating.
- **Diet:** Spicy food can irritate the back passage, especially if it's trying to heal from an infection or sore. Avoid strong spicy foods like curries, hot peppers and chillies.
- **Avoid constipation:** Constipation makes you strain to pass a stool and will aggravate (or even cause) problems like haemorrhoids and anal fissures. Haemorrhoids and fissures both cause intense pain in the back passage.
- **Anal fissures:** These 'splits' in the skin can be treated using olive oil (to relieve pain), tea tree oil (to promote healing and discourage infection – beware, it may sting at first), or fresh lemon juice (to dull the pain, although it may also sting when you first apply it).
- **Haemorrhoids:** Witch hazel compresses applied to an affected (external) area can reduce swelling and inflammation. Herbal pilewort ointment may be applied 2–3 times a day. Using a bidet with cold water may also help reduce haemorrhoid swellings. Medicinal preparations like Anusol are very effective at reducing haemorrhoid inflammation and easing pain.

- **Acute pain:** This can be helped by sitting on a rubber ring, or on a ring made using a towel rolled into a circle. This will help take the pressure off a sore anus or rectum when you are sitting.
- **Alternative treatments:** Colonic irrigation, while popular with many, should be avoided if there is *any* problem with the back passage. The same advice applies to anal intercourse or the insertion of foreign objects into the back passage.
- **Further information:**
  Self-care on familydoctor.org,
  http://familydoctor.org/flowcharts/527.html

Wind and Bloating

There are two major ways in which we produce gas. Firstly, we swallow air when we eat. Some people swallow more than others and certain foods (for example, aerated drinks) also contribute to this. Some people swallow air as a nervous reaction – called 'aerophagy' – and this can cause quite severe wind problems from both ends. Secondly, wind is a by-product of food digestion. Fats and proteins cause little gas, but carbohydrates (vegetables, beans, pulses, fruit, whole grains), sugars, dairy products and foods that contain sorbitol (often found in sugar-free items) all produce gas as they are digested. Lactose intolerance can also cause a lot of uncomfortable wind.

The digestive tract, in particular the large intestine, contains billions of bacteria – each of us has about 1 kilogram (2lb) in our body. Some of these, like various strains of *lactobacilli* and *bifidobacteria*, are very good for gut health. They benefit from the food that passes through our gut, while we benefit from their by-products – vitamins and other chemicals they produce, as well as the stimulation our immune systems need to function optimally. These 'good' bugs also keep potentially harmful bacteria such as the *Escherischia* (like *E. coli*) and *Streptococci* strains in check.

Contrary to popular belief, intestinal bacteria don't tend to create much gas as a by-product. In fact, they mostly consume it. Professor Glenn Gibson, a leading British researcher of gut flora, says that without bacteria, the average person would produce about 25 litres of gas every day. Thankfully, intestinal bacteria reduce this to approximately 5 litres. That's roughly 20–30 farts a day. Anyone who claims they don't break that much wind is either mistaken, doing it in their sleep – or lying! If you think 5 litres is bad enough, spare a thought for anyone suffering from the exceedingly rare disorder pneumatosis cystoides intestinalis; they have no intestinal bacteria to reduce the overall gas load and as a consequence they *do* produce around 25 litres of wind every day.

Bloating is often a consequence of wind – but not always. It can be the result of a sluggish bowel and come from feelings of fullness, perhaps due to constipation or overeating. A full bladder, water retention or pregnancy can also cause bloating. In some people, a high-fibre diet can cause bloating, while in others it may relieve it. Wind and bloating are also associated with moderately troublesome conditions like gastritis, IBS, malabsorption and parasitic infections.

Bloating occasionally indicates serious abdominal problems like bowel tumours or Crohn's disease, and two rare emergency conditions, peritonitis and intestinal obstruction. However, in these cases bloating will virtually always be accompanied by other serious symptoms – acute pain, diarrhoea, bleeding and so on.

Self-Help for Wind and Bloating

- **Diet:** Look at your eating and drinking habits and try and identify areas that you can modify to reduce your 'gas intake'. Try the following:
  - Eat and drink more slowly. This reduces the amount of air you'll swallow.
  - Try to identify and cut out foods that give you wind. Some foods are notorious for their gassiness – onions (especially fried), baked beans, whole grains and 'vegetarian' diets. Other causes are not so well known; fructose, not only present in fruit juices and drinks, but also found in wheat and artichokes, can increase your gas load.
  - Avoid dairy foods if you think you may be lactase deficient. The enzyme lactase is necessary to digest lactose (milk sugar) properly and some people – mostly those of Mediterranean, African, Asian and Native American heritage – don't always produce enough lactase, with the result that undigested milk sugars ferment within the gut, producing wind. Lactase supplements can help in these situations.

- Starches – with the exception of rice and rice flour – produce gas when broken down in the intestine. Use rice instead of potato or wheat-based carbohydrates.
- Avoid chewing gum and sucking hard sweets as they make you swallow more often (as does smoking).
- Avoid sorbitol-based sweeteners and products containing sorbitol – they can be found in sugar-free products like mints, for instance.

- **See your dentist:** Badly fitting dentures encourage air to be swallowed, so get your dentures checked if they feel loose.
- **'Anti-gas' preparations:** Remedies containing simethicone – for example, Rennie Deflatine, Setlers Wind-eze®, Maalox (various types) and Mylanta II (US) – help by combining small wind bubbles in the stomach that are then more easily burped up. (Note that some of these products, for instance, Remegel Wind Relief, also contain sorbitol – see above.) Activated charcoal tablets can help reduce colon wind, and Beano® (available in the US) may help digest the sugars found in beans and many vegetables, thereby reducing gas.
- **Herbal help:** Celery seeds can help reduce wind, as can fresh dill tea (simply brew some fresh dill in boiling water for a few minutes, strain and drink). Peppermint oil also helps prevent wind.
- **Homeopathy:** Lycopodium, arsenicum and argentum nitricum are all recommended for relief of wind and bloating.
- **If all else fails:** It may sound like a joke but it isn't – you can buy special airtight underwear (Under-Ease) from the US that contains a replaceable charcoal filter designed to remove the unsociable smells associated with troublesome and persistent wind – visit www.under-tec.com or call (1) 888 433 5913 for details (from outside the US call (1) 719 584 7782).
- **Further Information:**
  National Digestive Diseases Information Clearinghouse,
  www.niddk.nih.gov/health/digest/pubs/gas/gas.htm

Urgency, Frequency and Incomplete Evacuation

'I was in the bar, having a drink, and I suddenly sensed an ominous feeling. I knew I had a matter of seconds to make it to the loo, and a whole crowded bar to get through. Barging past people was bad enough, but as I burst through the door to the Ladies' Room, I saw a row of girls staring at me, arms folded, waiting their turn. I didn't have time to queue up, but I couldn't think what to say either. As soon as I saw a door to a cubicle open, I pushed forward, apologizing, and slammed the cubicle door shut behind me. I was already a bit too late and my embarrassment at having been caught short was only made ten times worse when I heard all the gossiping and tut-tutting going on outside.'

Andrea, 23, who suffers from ulcerative colitis (feelings of urgency are a common feature of this disorder)

'Urgency' means that desperate rush to the bathroom that often happens when we have an attack of holiday diarrhoea. Most of us, most of the time, manage to make it to the loo, but sometimes we don't and the resulting embarrassment and feeling of shame can be dreadful – even when nobody else knows what's happened. Bowel control is something that, because it's learned when we are toddlers, seems to remain firmly embedded in our minds as an essential ingredient of being 'grown up'. Anyone who can't control their bowels is immediately open to ridicule – how can anyone fail to control something so basic, something even *toddlers* can do?

'Frequency' refers to the need to empty our bowels more often than normal – another symptom often associated with irritated intestines. Increased frequency is often accompanied by feelings that the bowel has not been emptied properly – what doctors refer to as 'incomplete evacuation'. Most people open their bowels a maximum of 2–3 times a day, but if you have severe frequency and urgency you can find yourself going to the loo 10, 15 or even 20 times a day.

What Causes These Problems?

The number of conditions that may cause these symptoms is relatively small. The most common cause is haemorrhoids. Proctitis and IBS are two other common causes of feelings of urgency, frequency and incomplete evacuation. Less commonly, such symptoms may be caused by ulcerative colitis, Crohn's disease and (even more rarely) bowel and anal cancer.

Self-Help for Urgency, Frequency and Incomplete Evacuation

■ 'Can't Wait' cards: These credit-card-sized cards are available from associations like National Association for Colitis and Crohn's Disease (NACC) and are designed for people who often need to find a toilet fast. They state that the holder of the card is suffering from a non-contagious condition that causes them to need the toilet urgently. Can't Wait cards can spare you the embarrassment of having to ask and explain, and give your request more credibility. Use them in shops and offices, aircraft or public places.

■ **Go prepared:** If urgency is a persistent feature of your daily life, then be prepared. Carry a spare change of underwear, or wear a discreet incontinence pad (even a feminine pad) in your underpants in case of emergencies.

■ **Don't rely on public toilets:** You might be lucky enough to get to a public toilet, only to discover with horror that it has no toilet paper. Always carry a handy pack of tissues with you, just in case, and a small packet of wet wipes.

■ **Identify your triggers:** Some people find certain things act as triggers – try to identify what yours are. Stress often acts as a laxative and specific foods like coffee (caffeine), chocolate and alcohol can too. It could be that certain times of day are worse than others – morning is often a bad time for many people. Learn what your triggers are and then work around them.

■ **Avoid smoking:** Ask any smoker what gets them to the bathroom to open their bowels and invariably they'll tell you it's the first cigarette of the day. Nicotine exerts immensely powerful effects on the body, one of these being a laxative one. If you were ever going to quit smoking, now is the time.

■ **Strengthen your pelvic floor:** The muscles of the pelvic floor are structured somewhat like a figure '8', running from back to front – from the anus to the vagina (in girls) or scrotum (in boys). They support our internal abdominal organs and help control the bowel and bladder sphincters. If you have urgency problems, it is very important that these muscles are toned. You can do pelvic floor exercises discreetly at any time. Just gently squeeze and tighten the muscles, as if you're pulling up and in, hold and then relax. You can do it in stages, pulling up a little bit at a time, and holding in between. You can do them standing or sitting, and regular practice (several times daily) is essential.

■ **Frequency problems:** These can be lessened by avoiding any foods that act as laxatives or stimulants – like caffeine, alcohol and spicy, rich or fatty foods.

■ **Relaxation:** Relaxation calms the digestive system and can be useful if your problems are aggravated by stress – as they often are with IBS and even some of the inflammatory conditions like ulcerative colitis and Crohn's disease.

There *may* be some element of mind–over–matter when it comes to controlling urgency and frequency.

■ Herbal help: Valerian has a calming effect on the digestive system.

Itchy Bottom

The skin around our anus is sensitive – one only has to see what happens to a baby whose nappy has been left unchanged for even a little while to see how sensitive it is. When we get diarrhoea, the resulting faeces are generally more acidic than a normal stool, so it's quite normal for our skin to get sore. And sore skin can get itchy.

Children are prone to getting an 'itchy bum' because they're not always careful to wipe themselves properly after going to the loo. Itching isn't always caused by lapses in hygiene, although if you have a bowel problem – perhaps IBS, haemorrhoids or an anal fissure – being scrupulously clean is even more important.

In children, the commonest cause of an itchy bottom is threadworm infection, while among adults it is most often due to haemorrhoids or pruritus ani. Eczema and excessive sweating can also cause an itchy bottom (it's also common for people to get dry, itchy and sensitive skin as they get older). Proctitis and anal fissures may also cause this irritating symptom, as can anal cancer – though this is very rare.

Self-Help for an Itchy Bottom

■ Hygiene: Keeping skin clean and dry helps relieve anal itching. Make sure you wear loose, cotton underwear to prevent overheating and sweating, which make itching worse.

■ Hands: Especially with children, keep fingernails short to avoid scratching the skin, and wash hands regularly.

■ Skin creams: Itching may be caused – or aggravated – by dry skin. Keep your skin well moisturized, but avoid strong soaps or toiletries that irritate or dry your skin out. For delicate skin near the anus, only use unperfumed moisturizers. Olive oil is a good natural choice.

- **Ayurvedic medicine:** The nut Anacardium orientale produces a bitter black juice that can help itchy skin, especially if it's caused by haemorrhoids. People who like dairy products are normally said to respond well to this treatment.
- **Herbal help:** It is claimed that devil's claw relieves itchy skin that has no clear cause, and aloe vera (gel, applied locally) and chamomile (applied as a compress, or in a cream) also offer relief.

CHAPTER 3

How to Get the Best from your Doctor

Overcoming Shyness

There's little argument that bowel problems represent the last taboo in today's world. Forty years ago, women died in their thousands because they were too embarrassed to go to their doctor with a breast lump. Today, there are fashion shows promoting breast cancer research, with supermodels happily waving the flag. Thank goodness that they do – as a result there are thousands of women alive today playing with grandchildren they thought they would never see.

Unfortunately, sufferers of bowel disease stand almost in the same place as breast cancer victims did four decades ago. It may not be embarrassing to talk about your stomach ulcer, but what about telling friends that blood and diarrhoea are squirting out of your bottom, or that you have terrible wind and problems with incontinence? Not many people would.

It's one thing not to want to make coffee morning conversation about your bowels, but many thousands of people are too shy even to tell their doctor and they quite literally end up dying ... of embarrassment.

'I couldn't face telling anyone. I kept it to myself for over a year before I told my husband I had chronic diarrhoea. Eventually, I plucked up courage to go to the doctor, but I was a nervous wreck by the time I got there. I was, and still am, very embarrassed talking about bodily functions. I only recently discovered that bowel problems run in our family, and that my younger brother was also diagnosed with ulcerative colitis – like I now have been – some time ago. If only I knew, I would have seen the doctor much earlier.'
Ellie, age 29

Picking the Right Words

It's possibly the hardest place to start – what words do you use? Most people find medical terminology (like 'stools', 'flatus', 'anus') ugly and uncomfortable to use, while the other words we know about are either too babyish ('poo', 'number twos') or too crude ('fart', 'shit', 'arse'). However, if you use vague descriptions like 'down there' or 'down below' in order to avoid mentioning these embarrassing words your doctor can become confused about what you're really trying to say.

There's no easy answer, but it helps if you realize that doctors hear 'embarrassing' words all the time and aren't generally fazed by any of them. If they sense your embarrassment, they will often step in to help – one gastroenterologist I know often uses words like 'shit', knowing that he can break the ice this way. If knowing your doctor isn't going to be offended doesn't help, then tell him you are embarrassed about having to discuss the subject with him and usually he or she will help you along in an effort to spare your blushes.

The following useful phrases are both descriptive yet not too awkward for anyone who feels uncomfortable discussing intimate body parts and functions with their doctor:

'BELCHING' (BURPING) AND 'SOUTHERLY WIND' (FARTING)

Most people normally say 'burping' or 'belching' and neither of these words is likely to offend. When it comes to 'farting', however, there may be sensitivities – even though the word is so commonly used that it may soon carry no social stigma at all. Some people like to refer to farting as 'southerly wind', but if you think this is too twee, another option is simply to call it 'breaking wind'. If you're asked to be even more specific you can always add 'from the back end'.

'NAUSEA' AND 'VOMITING'

Bear in mind there is a difference between these two words – nausea normally means feelings of sickness, whereas vomiting means actually throwing up. You can feel 'nauseous', but this doesn't generally mean you've been physically sick. If you have, you should always tell your doctor you have 'vomited'.

'BACK PASSAGE'

'Back passage' is a very useful phrase – it means the rectum and anus. 'Tail-end' is another useful description normally understood as meaning the buttocks, anus or anal region.

'OPENING THE BOWELS'

This means 'passing a stool' (another reasonable phrase), or having a poo. If you're constipated you can say you have been 'trying unsuccessfully' or 'repeatedly' to open your bowels.

FEELINGS OF 'URGENCY' OR 'FREQUENCY'

'Urgency' indicates that rush to the loo that we often get with severe diarrhoea, while 'frequency' means the need to visit the bathroom much more often than normal.

'NOT QUITE MAKING IT ON TIME', BEING 'CAUGHT SHORT', 'LEAKAGE' AND 'WET WIND'

Essentially, these phrases refer to incontinence – although 'leakage' can also be used if you're trying to explain mucus discharge or bleeding from your bottom. 'Wet wind' is a good phrase to explain the sort of leakage that sometimes happens when passing wind.

UNABLE TO PASS A STOOL 'SATISFACTORILY' OR 'COMFORTABLY', FEELINGS OF 'INCOMPLETE EVACUATION'

These two phrases can be used to help describe the discomfort caused by haemorrhoids, anal fissures or even severe diarrhoea, or the feeling that there's 'more to come' when we've opened our bowels.

For Children

Some parents encourage their children to use words like 'vagina', 'penis' and 'anus' at an early age; others feel they sound somewhat awkward coming from a youngster's mouth and prefer them to use words more suited to children. Little girls often use the terms 'front bottom' and 'back bottom' to differentiate between urinary and bowel problems. With boys there is only one 'bottom', which makes life a little simpler. When you're taking a child to the doctors, use whatever terms your child normally uses and, if necessary, add a few adult specifics to help clarify things.

Cultural and Other Differences

Doctors see hundreds of patients every week and they're all different. Some patients are very shy and have difficulty expressing their problems; others are hilariously frank. Some patients, often the elderly, are quite embarrassed about being examined by a doctor of the opposite sex. People living in certain cultures find various forms of nudity degrading or contrary to their religious beliefs. Asian women, for example, traditionally cover their legs, upper body and upper arms, and may find hospital gowns uncomfortably revealing. Asian men, by contrast, cover themselves from the waist to the knees and even in the presence of other men they may find nakedness humiliating. Some religions consider all body secretions to be unclean or polluting and people may not only have difficulty discussing them, but may need to observe religious rituals with respect to cleansing – for example, they may need running water (as opposed to bathing) to wash themselves in hospital. In addition, some cultures view medicines in a way that may not be known to the doctor: for instance, the notion of taking pills as a preventative measure is not always readily accepted, and having a stoma is hugely stigmatized in some communities.

This is not a trivial point when it comes to digestive health: according to a health survey of minority groups, Bangladeshi, Irish and Indian men suffer more with long-term digestive problems compared to the general population. The same is true for women of Pakistani, Bangladeshi and Irish origin.

When it comes to health, people are embarrassed and uncommunicative for a whole host of reasons – and doctors are not mind readers. Don't assume your doctor will automatically know, for example, that you are shy about him examining your body. If you are, tell him. If you are scared to talk about your problem for fear that it is serious, let him know up-front. Get your doctor on your side by telling him how you feel. One honest exchange can spare a dozen embarrassing moments.

Summary

- Doctors generally understand you may be embarrassed talking about digestive problems – but don't let this prevent you telling them if you feel awkward.
- Use words that are descriptive but cause you least embarrassment.
- If you would rather be examined by a doctor of the same sex, request one.
- If you feel better having a friend or relative with you, take them to the consultation with you.
- If your teenager feels embarrassed by you being there, let them talk to the doctor alone. Obviously it is not appropriate or desirable for younger children to go alone.
- If your culture or religion makes certain things like physical examinations uncomfortable, tell your doctor.
- Explain your views and thoughts about certain procedures and medicines, especially if they differ from those your doctor may expect to encounter.

Go Prepared

Be Organized

Doctors make their diagnoses on the basis of symptoms. However, different people with the same illness may present with different symptoms. It can be a minefield – for both you and your doctor. So before your visit it's a good idea to sit down and think about the questions that your doctor may ask you. These include:

- What are your exact symptoms?
- When did they start?
- Are they the same, or have they changed at all?
- Are they getting worse?
- How severe are they? If you're bleeding, for example, is the blood dripping into the toilet every time you pass a stool, or is it a small bright red streak that is just visible on the toilet paper?
- Have you been travelling – especially to exotic or undeveloped countries?
- Is anything different in your lifestyle – e.g. stress, your work pattern or job, are you eating different food, taking medicines, or have you had a tummy bug or other illness?

- Is there anything else you believe is relevant, or may be connected?

Have an Agenda

It is also important to think about *what you want* out of the consultation. Try to identify the questions that you would like answered – for example, do you want to know if you could have a specific illness? Think about any worries and anxieties that you might want addressed. Are you worried that you have the same cancer that your aunt died from? Talk to the doctor about your fears, no matter how silly they may suddenly seem in the cold light of day. Perhaps you want reassurance, or you might want some tests done – whatever it is, make sure you say, otherwise the consultation may end up being frustrating and unsatisfying. It helps the doctor if he knows what is on your mind and what you would like to happen.

Be Up-front

Sexuality nowadays occupies the foreground of most people's lives, as well as the front pages of the popular media, and there is little shame in discussing sexual preferences and activities today. Anyone who indulges in anal intercourse, whether male or female, is at higher risk than normal of contracting anal and rectal infections, conditions or even injuries that may need medical treatment.

Don't make your doctor guess. Say if you've been fooling about with sex toys, if you're gay or if you engage in anal intercourse, or if your problem could be linked to (or affected by) your sex life. You're much more likely to get the appropriate treatment – and quicker – if you don't make your physician play detective.

Checklist for Doctor's Visit

Use the following checklist to make an accurate list of your symptoms.

Constipation:

When was the last time you opened your bowels?

What are your stools like? Describe them.

Diarrhoea:

How many times a day is it happening?

How does this compare with your normal habit?

Do you get desperate urges to go to the loo and have you been incontinent?

Have you travelled abroad recently?

Bleeding:

Does it happen regularly and when did it start?

Does it happen when you open your bowels?

Do you have pain when you open your bowels?

Are there streaks of bright red blood on the toilet tissue, is it mixed in with your stools, or is it dark in colour?

Wind:

Are you passing excessive gas?

Do you feel bloated or 'full'?

Do these feelings happen after meals?

Has your diet changed recently?

Pain:

Do you have abdominal or rectal pain?

How long have you had it?

Is it continuous, or does it only happen at specific times, for example when you try to pass a stool?

Itching:

Is it in one specific area of your body, for example your anal region?

Does it happen only at night, or is it more continuous?

Mucus:

Do you have mucus or any unusual or unpleasant-smelling discharge from your back passage?

Nausea and vomiting:

Do you feel or have you been sick?

Is it associated with certain times or activities, for example on waking in the morning or at mealtimes, or is it more constant?

Other questions:

Has your appetite changed recently?

Have you gained or lost weight unexpectedly?

Are you, or might you be, pregnant? When was the first day of your last period?

Do you feel unusually tired, lethargic, weak or dizzy?

Have you noticed anything else recently? For example, any hair loss that might be greater than normal or excessively dry skin?

Is it possible that sexual activities are playing even a minor role in your problem?

CHAPTER 4

Investigating the Problems – a Look at Tests, Scans and 'Scopes

There are many tests that may be done to pinpoint a specific bowel problem. Some of them are fine if you don't mind needles; others are fine if you don't mind a gloved finger fiddling about 'down there'. Many of us mind it greatly! Some tests, like endoscopies, may involve a sedative, which helps if you're nervous – although it does rather limit your ability to drive yourself home afterwards. Others – like ultrasound scans and some x-rays – are completely painless and simply involve you lying back and relaxing (supposedly). Here are the most common tests – how they are performed and their purposes...

Stool Tests

Stool specimens are asked for if the problem might be caused by infection – perhaps a bacterial infection like salmonella, or a parasitic infection like threadworms. If there are any bacteria or parasites, these will normally be present in the faeces.

Stool specimens may also show 'occult' bleeding – i.e. blood that cannot be visibly seen in the stools, but is present nonetheless. This may occur when there is bleeding higher up in the stomach or the upper reaches of the small intestine: by the time it is passed, it is no longer red, but dark brown or black and therefore may not be noticed.

Stool samples can also show increased amounts of mucus or pus, and will invariably show any blood that comes from the lower parts of the colon, rectum and anus.

Breath Tests

A simple analysis of the gas composition of exhaled breath is sometimes used to detect the presence of *Helicobacter pylori* in the stomach, or an overgrowth of bacteria in the small intestine.

Blood Tests

Blood is normally taken from a vein in the arm, using a fine needle with a syringe and a series of small vacuum tubes that 'suck' blood out automatically when they're popped into the syringe housing. You'll normally have a pressure cuff wrapped around your upper arm to increase the blood pressure and make collection easier, and you may also be asked to squeeze a small ball, or pump your hand into a fist. Apart from the slight scratch when the needle is put in, blood tests are not a problem for most people, but do tell the doctor or nurse if you are needle phobic, if you have one arm that gives blood more easily than the other, or if you have tricky veins.

The following list includes the various kinds of tests and the more common factors that doctors can study in blood, in order to understand what is going wrong.

- **Full blood count:** This is one of the most common tests. It measures the levels of basic components in the blood, the number of red blood cells, white blood cells and platelets. A reduced number of red blood cells or lower levels of haemoglobin may indicate, for example, anaemia, while an increase in the numbers of the various white blood cells may indicate an infection.
- **Erythrocyte sedimentation rate (ESR):** The ESR measures how quickly red blood cells settle at the bottom of a blood sample. If there is active inflammation, red blood cells tend to clump together, making them sink faster. A raised ESR can therefore indicate active inflammation.
- **C-reactive protein:** A raised level of C-reactive protein indicates there is inflammation. This test is often done in conjunction with the ESR.
- **Ferritin:** Low ferritin levels may indicate the need for iron supplements; the levels also vary when there is inflammation.
- **Vitamin B12 and folic acid:** Because vitamin B12 is only absorbed in the end portion of the ileum, anyone who has had severe damage to (or removal of)

the ileum may need regular Vitamin B12 injections. Low folic acid levels can indicate poor nutrition and perhaps poor absorption from the small intestine.

- **Liver function tests (LFTs):** Liver function can be affected by inflammatory bowel diseases (IBDs) and also by certain medication. LFTs also measure the levels of important proteins like albumin, which can be affected by poor nutrition or absorption.

- **Urea and electrolytes (U&E):** The levels of urea and creatinine, sodium, potassium, chloride and bicarbonate give an indication of how the kidneys are functioning. They also give clues about nutritional status – especially useful if you are being given extra fluids and salt because of severe diarrhoea.

- **Endomysial antibody (EMA) screening test:** This test looks for special antibodies in the blood which are always present in people with coeliac disease, but which are never found in people who don't have it.

- **Bone chemistry:** This test measures blood calcium, phosphate and levels of alkaline phosphatase, which helps doctors see how well nourished we are. It is also used to check for bone problems – though it doesn't give much information about the possibility of osteoporosis.

- **Magnesium:** Levels of magnesium can become very low with severe diarrhoea and can cause muscle weakness.

Scans

- **Ultrasound scans:** Using ultra-high frequency sound waves, these painless scans give internal pictures of the body's organs and can help doctors detect tissue masses, abscesses and fluid. They can also show thickened or inflamed sections of the intestines. A hand-held device rather like a microphone is covered in jelly and then gently moved around the surface of the abdomen to give two-dimensional black and white pictures of our insides on a monitor. Ultrasound scans normally take about 15–20 minutes. Endo-anal ultrasound scans use a probe placed just inside the anus, and are performed when there might be a problem with the sphincter muscle structure – for example, in people suffering with faecal incontinence.

- **CT scan (computerized tomography):** This uses an enormous round machine with a hole in the middle, through which the patient, lying on a table, slowly passes. The CT scanner takes multiple x-rays, which are like 'slices' of the patient. A computer then puts these together to recreate a three-dimensional image. You may have an intravenous injection of a special dye to show certain features up better, or you may swallow a contrast liquid or have it injected into the rectum. You normally have to fast for around 4 hours beforehand, and will need to stay still while the scan is performed. It can take 30–40 minutes. Newer machines are becoming much faster and advanced technology has also meant the development of spiral CT and 'multi-slice' CT scans, which are quicker.

- **PET scan (positron emission tomography):** This is one of the newest medical scanning techniques. It is often used to analyse the brain and heart, but can also detect tumours. PET scanning measures the uptake by certain body tissues of molecules like oxygen or glucose that are specially labelled with a radioactive substance. This indicates how well the body tissues are functioning. Tumours, for example, have a high energy demand and labelled glucose shows up clearly in a tumour. PET scans give more information about the activity of body tissues rather than their physical form.

- **MRI scan (magnetic resonance imaging):** MRI scans use magnetism (not x-rays) to create three-dimensional, very detailed pictures of the human body. They are very good for looking at solid objects like the bones and liver, though less good at the intestines, which are constantly moving. Patients lie on a table inside a small chamber of the scanner and although you don't feel anything, you hear a loud series of 'knocking' noises. People with claustrophobia may not be comfortable or able to tolerate an MRI scan while awake. Newer 'open' MRI scanners may minimize this problem.

- **Nuclear medicine (white cell) scan:** This technique can be useful for locating areas of inflammation in the intestines. A sample of blood is taken and the white cells are given a mildly radioactive 'marker' before being injected back into the patient. Because white cells are naturally attracted to areas of inflammation, they show up in concentration when the body is scanned using a gamma camera that picks up the radioactive marker. There are other types of nuclear medicine scan that use different radioactive isotopes.

X-rays

X-rays, perhaps one of the most common – and oldest – medical imaging techniques, give the doctor a 'snapshot' of the chest, abdomen or bones. In order for soft tissue such as the digestive tract to show up on the x-ray properly, a 'contrast' substance needs to be introduced. Contrast substances such as barium are swallowed, injected into the rectum or injected into the blood vessels.

- **Abdominal x-rays:** Abdominal radiography normally looks at the pattern of gas (wind) in the digestive tract – this can give a lot of information about what is happening inside the abdominal cavity. It can show intestinal obstructions and also give important clues to the extent and severity of diseases like UC. It does not normally involve a contrast element.
- **Joint radiography:** While bones aren't digestive organs, they can be affected by IBDs. Bone x-rays can show inflammation in the spine, joints, pelvis or hips.
- **Bone densitometry (DEXA scan):** If malnutrition has been a chronic problem, or if steroids have been taken for a significant period of time, there is always a chance that there is insufficient calcium stored in the bones – which may eventually lead to osteoporosis and bone fractures. DEXA scans check the density of bones in the lower spine and femur (thigh) bone and are often given to patients who suffer with UC or Crohn's.
- **Barium meal and barium swallow:** A barium meal involves swallowing a drink of liquid barium – a contrast medium that shows up the oesophagus, stomach and duodenum. It is normally used to highlight lesions. A barium swallow, or follow-through, is done to track the speed at which the liquid travels through the upper part of the digestive tract and small intestine.
- **Small bowel enema:** If really detailed pictures of the small intestine are needed, or if a barium follow-through has not produced satisfactory results, then a small bowel enema may be done. Here, barium and air are pumped directly into the small intestine through a fine tube that is passed down the oesophagus and stomach. It produces detailed pictures, but may be more uncomfortable than a barium swallow.
- **Barium enema:** Barium enemas give x-ray pictures of the large intestine. Barium and air are pumped into the rectum using a tube, and then an air-filled balloon is placed just inside the rectum to prevent the contents from slipping out (although they always feel as if they're just about to). Several x-rays are taken as the body is tipped to each side to move the barium into the right positions. Barium enemas are given on an empty colon, so you will be given drugs beforehand to empty your bowels – make sure you are not

far from a bathroom when this happens. After this test you will pass thick, clay-like stools that can be very difficult to flush away. The best tip is to empty your bowels as much as possible immediately after the x-ray while still in hospital. If you are still passing clay when you get home, tip a whole bucket of water down the toilet immediately after you flush, to help move the barium. And don't worry – your stools will soon return to normal.

Endoscopies

- **Gastroscopy:** This is generally done if the doctor needs to see the stomach lining and take a small tissue sample (biopsy) to test for infections like *Helicobacter pylori* or confirm a diagnosis of gastritis. It is also done if blood has been reported in the vomit or stools, if it has shown up in a faecal occult blood (FOB) test, or if you have symptoms that include weight loss and extreme tiredness (especially if you are over 50). The gastroscope tube is inserted into the stomach by swallowing; you will be given an anaesthetic spray to numb the back of your throat and possibly a sedative if you feel nervous or uncomfortable about the procedure.
- **Proctoscopy:** This is normally a quick procedure, and only involves looking at the first few centimetres of the anal canal. It is often used to check for fistulas, internal haemorrhoids and internal prolapse.
- **Sigmoidoscopy:** Sigmoidoscopes, which are either rigid or flexible, are inserted into the bowel through the anus and can be used to look higher up in the colon, usually up to about 60cm (24in) inside. Rigid sigmoidoscopies – often done in outpatient clinics – can show how severe a case of UC might be. Flexible sigmoidoscopies are usually done on an empty bowel, normally without sedation, although most doctors will oblige if you feel very nervous about the procedure being done to you. Because air is pumped into the colon to open up the bowel for a better view, it can be an uncomfortable procedure, especially if you already have abdominal tenderness or pain.
- **Colonoscopy:** The 'king' of bowel endoscopy procedures, a colonscopy allows a good view of the entire large bowel and the end of the small intestine (the terminal ileum). It can be used to accurately assess UC and Crohn's disease, as well as any suture joins that have been made during surgery. Laxatives are normally given beforehand to clear out the colon, and the procedure is done on an inpatient or day-case basis. Because sedation is used, it is often less

uncomfortable than some other 'scope tests that don't offer sedation (like barium enemas).

The Future of Diagnostic Tests

Scientists are continually trying to make medical examinations less uncomfortable for the patient and more detailed for the doctor. Conventional imaging tests often fail to spot the source of intestinal bleeding because they can't see the entire length of the gut. Upper endoscopies can only see down as far as the first third of the small intestine, while colonoscopies can only see up to the last metre (3–4ft) or so of small intestine. Because the small intestine is 5–6 metres (15–20ft) long, this leaves a 2–3 metre (5–10ft) section in the middle that cannot normally be seen at all.

One of the newest innovations is a tiny camera-in-a-capsule which gives extraordinarily accurate pictures of the intestinal tract. Containing a battery, light source, radio transmitter and camera, the capsule (the size of a large multivitamin tablet) transmits pictures of the intestines to a wireless recorder the patient wears on a belt. After swallowing the capsule, the patient carries on as normal while the images are collected, then, 6–8 hours later, the pictures are downloaded onto a computer for the doctor to view. Preliminary trials of capsule-camera devices already indicate a high degree of success in locating gastrointestinal bleeding.

Recent work conducted by a team at the Ludwig Institute for Cancer Research, New York Branch at Memorial Sloan-Kettering, shows that the way the immune system reacts to specific tumour markers (antigens) may eventually offer an opportunity for doctors to detect bowel cancer. By identifying which of these antigens is produced by bowel cancers and then identifying any antibodies to them in blood samples, doctors may find a quick and reliable method for detecting bowel cancers at very early stages. Work continues on identifying more of the specific colon cancer antigens (about a dozen are known so far).

Diagnosis – or Is It?

Finding the Cause

Normally, we visit our doctor and, during the consultation or after a few basic tests, he or she uncovers the problem and recommends an appropriate treatment. Most of the time, the process is straightforward. But not always. Many bowel symptoms may be vague, or apply to several potential causes. It is therefore quite common for your doctor not to immediately get to the root of your problem – they often need to eliminate the most likely causes first.

Because today's scientists can clone animals and genetically select embryos, it is tempting to believe that doctors should be able to spot every medical problem, quickly and accurately. I'm not an apologist for poor medicine, but neither are doctors superhuman. They can't – too often because of limited medical or financial resources – assume that every case of constipation is caused by bowel cancer and send every patient for a full screen of exhaustive tests. There will inevitably be an occasional patient whose serious problems weren't spotted early enough.

However, doctors should NEVER rule out the possibility of you having a rare disorder simply because it *is* rare and statistically unlikely to happen in their catchment area. If your doctor does rule out a problem simply on the grounds of rarity, question him. Ask him to explain his logic and make sure that he tests for *all* eventualities once the common causes have been eliminated.

A patient's job is to help the doctor isolate their problem as quickly as possible, by giving him or her the best quality information. Equally, your doctor is obliged (at least morally) to give you a satisfactory explanation of what he thinks your problem may be, and tell you what he proposes to do.

You are entitled to ask questions. You are entitled to know about the medicines you are prescribed – what they are supposed to do, how long you will need to take them, what the chances are of them working and what the side effects may be. Your doctor may not always know the answers, but you are also entitled to ask him about self-help measures you might be able to try and also about alternative therapies.

Most doctors are pushed for time, but if your questions are focused and precise, and you go prepared, you can still get all the relevant information in a fairly brief session. If your doctor tells you he doesn't have the time to answer all your questions, book another, longer, appointment. A doctor who doesn't have time to explain the essential basics to his patients is not doing his job properly. Remember, it's your body – not his. If you are still dissatisfied with the diagnosis (or lack of one), or your problem persists or worsens, then you should feel completely comfortable about taking further action.

You must always go back to your doctor if:

- your problem doesn't respond to treatment within a reasonable time
- your symptoms change
- your problem gets worse

If you're still unhappy, seek a second opinion. There doesn't have to be war over it – doctors know their patients' rights. All you need to do is explain you feel there may be more to your problem than he seems happy to acknowledge and that you want to see someone else.

Summary

- Give your doctor the fullest and most accurate information you can.
- Be aware that sometimes your doctor will need to eliminate a few possibilities before reaching a diagnosis.
- Don't be afraid to ask for specific tests if you are worried and want to check you don't have a certain illness.
- Always tell your doctor if a particular medical condition runs in your family.
- Don't be afraid to ask questions. It's your body and you have the right to look after it.
- Remember – most health problems are caused by common and easily treated conditions, BUT rare illnesses can and do happen. Don't let your doctor rule out an illness simply because it is rare.
- Always request another opinion if you are dissatisfied.

Trying Alternatives

...And Getting your Doctor on your Side

People are increasingly turning to alternative and complementary therapies, for many reasons. Some want to take more control of their health and well-being and seeking complementary therapies is a useful way to do this. Some believe greatly in the power of 'natural' remedies and want to try to heal themselves with as little recourse to man-made drugs as possible. Some may be slightly distrustful of the medical profession, for any of a number of reasons, while others still may just want to check all avenues and explore all possibilities for an effective remedy to their problem.

Doctors are well aware that people want to try alternative and complementary therapies. Some of these – like osteopathy – are now accepted in mainstream medicine, while many more – acupuncture, homoeopathy, herbal medicine – are gaining good reputations among orthodox medical practitioners. However, health fraud and quackery do exist, and doctors are often genuinely concerned that their patients don't jeopardize their health by shunning a proven course of treatment in favour of an unproven and potentially dangerous alternative.

Dr Stuart Gould, Consultant Gastroenterologist at Epsom General Hospital, expresses a view shared by many: 'Doctors do realize that there is a strong desire to try complementary therapies among patients. But sometimes patients are scared to talk to their doctor about these – and when they are nervous, it's quite common for the words to come out all wrong. We don't want to see them abandon proven medicine in favour of something which may amount to nothing, but many doctors are normally quite happy to let them try some of the therapies that might help, even if they just relax the patient.'

As a patient, you may have to sell alternatives to your doctor. Tell them that you are keen to try the treatment *they* are suggesting and ask if they think it would conflict with the alternative therapy *you* want to try. Many complementary therapies have a good overall press and are unlikely to make your doctor defensive.

However, you may find your doctor is against some practices – for example, colonic irrigation (also called colonic hydrotherapy). From a medical perspective, there is a small risk of the bowel becoming perforated if the therapy is administered incorrectly, or if there is an underlying problem that might make the bowel wall liable to rupture. There have been (very) occasional incidences of infection and the treatment also has strong erotic associations – which don't normally underpin accepted medical practices. However, when done properly, it is extremely safe.

Research the treatments you are interested in, read up on what both the converts and the sceptics say and make your own decision. A simple Internet search will normally find any number of websites promoting alternative and complementary treatments. (I tend to view any website which both advocates and sells a particular therapy or product with a pinch of salt, as it has a vested financial interest in only speaking positively about it.) A visit to Quackwatch (www.quackwatch.org) or a related association, the National Council Against Health Fraud (www.ncahf.org/) may also provide you with some interesting counterpoints.

the medical
possibilities

—

The digestive system is made up of hollow organs like the stomach and colon, and solid ones like the liver. This book concentrates on disorders of the hollow digestive organs, particularly those in the lower part of the digestive tract, namely the small and large intestines – although I have for completeness included some key stomach disorders.

For what is essentially a hollow tube, the digestive tract is surprisingly complex. And the more complex anything is, the more that can go wrong with it. All sorts of factors can affect the digestive system – the way we live, the amount of stress we have, the food we eat, the infections we're exposed to, our genetic inheritance... Even health problems in other parts of the body can have a profound impact on gut health. This section of the book takes a closer look at the major factors that can affect our digestive system, what causes them and what we can do to stay healthy. It also examines what happens when we need hospital treatment.

CHAPTER 5

How Lifestyle Can Affect the Digestive System

We all know that the way we live affects our bodies. Most people readily recognize that partying too wildly and drinking too much alcohol will probably upset our stomachs – just as stress, tension and worry can cause tightly-knotted feelings or butterflies in the pit of our stomachs, or even nausea and vomiting. Yet other lifestyle choices – like how often and how vigorously we exercise – can also profoundly affect our digestive systems. Perhaps this fact is less well-known, although anyone who has trained for a marathon will probably know all about 'runner's trots'.

Our lifestyle affects our guts in a wide variety of ways – from a lack of routine causing a case of 'holiday constipation', a course of antibiotics giving us diarrhoea, or a case of stress-induced stomach ache. This section looks at the various effects of lifestyle on the digestive system and how we can make the best everyday choices for a healthy gut.

Drinking Too Much Alcohol

We've all enjoyed a wild night of partying – and most of us have also lived to regret it the next day. Drinking too much alcohol, particularly beer, can cause diarrhoea, although this generally eases off quickly and rarely lasts for more than a few hours. Alcohol irritates the stomach lining causing 'gastric irritation' and sometimes bleeding, especially when taken in large quantities or very frequently. Long-term alcohol abuse can result in cirrhosis, which destroys liver tissue. Cirrhosis is irreversible.

Who can it affect? Anyone of (supposedly) legal drinking age, although young teenagers and even pre-teens are increasingly among today's casualties.

Incidence: Common

Age–bias: None. However, the body's ability to break down large quantities of alcohol (and other toxins) does decrease with old age. In young people and children, the liver may simply not be developed enough to cope with large amounts of any toxin.

Risk factors:
- Liver disease can reduce the efficiency of the liver in metabolizing alcohol. Liver disease can be caused by infections such as hepatitis.
- People who are susceptible to ulcers or who have a history of digestive problems are more likely to suffer.
- Smokers or people suffering stress are more at risk of gastric irritation.

Symptoms caused by excess alcohol:
- Diarrhoea
- Headache
- Nausea
- Dehydration
- Stomach pains
- Feeling mentally 'blurry'
- Memory loss
- 'Coffee grounds' in the vomit can indicate that there has been some bleeding in the stomach.
- If the bleeding has been going on for a long time, you may feel tired and look pale and anaemic.
- If (rarely) sudden and massive bleeding occurs, you may feel faint, dizzy, short of breath and have abdominal pain or diarrhoea. Shock can follow, causing a rapid pulse, lowered blood pressure and pallor. **This is a medical emergency, seek medical help urgently.**

What can you do?

- Prevention is better than cure – avoid 'binge-drinking' or regular, heavy drinking.
- Pace yourself – over a long social evening, have two soft drinks for every one alcoholic drink.
- If you have ulcers you may be warned off alcohol altogether – If so, follow the advice.
- As alcohol causes dehydration, it is important to increase your (non-alcoholic!) fluid intake after a heavy night on the tiles.
- If your drinking is starting to cause problems (in work, relationships and so on), you may need to seek professional help for alcohol abuse.
- See Self-Help for Diarrhoea (page 14)

Stress

Stress seems to be an integral part of today's lifestyle – little wonder really when we're trying to juggle life, work, children, partners … Stress – along with fear, worry and tension – is a negative emotional state that can create sensations of pain in the body. Our guts are very closely linked to our emotions: upset children, for instance, often complain of 'tummy aches'. Adrenaline, which surges through the body as a physical response to fear, directly affects the intestines – in extreme cases, it can make the intestinal muscles contract to the point where the body expels waste ('I was shitting myself with fear'). Anxiety also prompts excess stomach acid to be produced, which can cause heartburn or aggravate existing ulcers. We can be 'sick with worry', and have 'butterflies in our stomach' when we're excited.

Who can it affect? Anyone. The International Stress Management Association (UK) says that in surveys 70 per cent of British adults report stress at work and about 30 per cent of those interviewed found balancing home and work life stressful.

Incidence: Extremely common.

Age-bias: None, although stress-related symptoms are possibly seen more frequently in adults aged between 20 and 40 years of age.

Risk factors:

■ People with Generalized Anxiety Disorders (GAD) and panic attacks may be more likely to experience abdominal pains, as are people in situations of emotional upheaval – for example, moving house, getting divorced, sitting exams, bereavement, a new job.

■ People with high-stress jobs, students, and adults struggling to cope with the demands of a job and family.

■ However, everyone feels stress and although we deal with it in our way, we are all at risk.

Common symptoms:

■ Diarrhoea

■ Abdominal pains

■ Nausea

■ Loss of appetite

■ Feelings of panic

■ Inability to sleep properly

■ Headaches

■ Red blotchy patches on the skin, especially on the chest and throat

■ Panic attacks

What can you do?

■ Identify the cause of the anxiety and try to relax. It's easier said than done, but important. Good relaxation techniques include:
  ■ Yoga
  ■ Deep breathing and/or meditation
  ■ Having a long hot bath
  ■ Taking a long walk outside
  ■ Exercise
  Whatever method you choose, make sure it fits with your lifestyle and personality. There are plenty of stress-relieving systems to choose from – if watching a good movie rather than exercising works for you, that's fine.

■ Try to retain your sense of humour and remember that today's strife will probably seem far less important in a week's time.

■ Antacid preparations can help people who may be overproducing stomach acid.

- Flower remedies and herbal help: Rescue Remedy is useful for easing panic or anxiety, as is the herb valerian.
- See your doctor if you are feeling overwhelmed.
- See Self-Help for Nausea (page 17), Diarrhoea (page 14), and Abdominal Pain (page 24).

Athlete's Diarrhoea

Athletes, and especially runners, often get what is known as 'runner's trots'. Though the repeated shaking of the body during running contributes to the problem, it is not the only cause. During exercise, up to 80 per cent of the digestive system's blood supply is diverted to help our muscles perform. This leaves less blood available to absorb nutrients from the gut that are released in digestion. In turn (and by osmosis), the unabsorbed nutrients attract more water into our guts, with the net effect that a watery slurry is quickly shaken down through our guts. The result: diarrhoea.

Who can it affect? Athlete's diarrhoea is a well-known curse of the long-distance runner, but can as easily happen to amateurs as professionals. It's a well-known phenomenon among marathon runners, but can affect shorter-distance runners like track athletes, as well as cyclists and anyone exercising vigorously.

Incidence: Common. As many as 50 per cent of all endurance athletes are affected by some form of gastric disturbance.

Age-bias: None known.

Symptoms: Diarrhoea. Because this happens in conjunction with physical exertion, dehydration can quickly set in.

Risk factors: Food intolerance or any other condition (like ulcerative colitis or Crohn's disease) that already predisposes you to diarrhoea will amplify any effects you might get through exercise alone. If you avoid drinking before a race and become dehydrated, it can make it worse.

What can you do?

- Take an anti-diarrhoeal preparation (like loperamide) before you start your run. Don't overdo it – follow dosage instructions.
- Watch what you eat:
  - Eliminate foods that normally cause you to have loose bowel movements.
  - Cut down on high-fibre foods beforehand.
  - Eliminate caffeine from your diet and have no more than 300mg of vitamin C in any supplements you take – these may cause or exacerbate diarrhoea. Some 'sports' drinks contain a lot of caffeine and possibly vitamin C, so read labels carefully.
  - Avoid new foods and supplements before a race – stick to those that you've 'tried and tested'.
  - Bananas are good and easily digested; so is white toast and jam or low-fibre cereal. Too much fruit, a fatty fry-up or a bowl of high-fibre cereal are not such a good idea!
- Stay well hydrated, and get used to jogging after drinking water – your stomach will soon become accustomed to the uneasy sensation.
- Go to the toilet before you start exercising.
- Increase your training gradually – sudden increases in intensity or endurance are more likely to cause diarrhoea.
- If the possibility of being 'caught short' makes you feel insecure, wear sponges or incontinence pads in your track shorts.
- Calm down: the gastrointestinal tract is extremely sensitive to stress. If you feel nervous, your bowels are likely to be twitchy, too.
- If you feel something 'coming on', slow your pace right down, take some deep, slow breaths and concentrate on squeezing your pelvic floor muscles. Mind over matter can help.
- See Self-Help for Diarrhoea (page 14).

Further information:
Cool Running Australia, www.coolrunning.com.au
Runner's World Magazine, www.runnersworld.com

Changes in Routine

Travelling, not being able to find a loo, or being reluctant to use public toilets are common experiences and ones that can easily disrupt your bowel habits. Changes in regular routine commonly lead to constipation.

Who can it affect? Anyone.

Incidence: Extremely common.

Age-bias: None, although children are often easily affected.

Symptoms: Constipation. This can lead to bloating and abdominal discomfort – and can also make you sluggish and grumpy.

What can you do?
- Try to make time in your day for your bowel habits whenever your routine is disrupted, or take additional measures (like adding a bulking agent to your daily diet) to prevent constipation from setting in.
- If you're abroad, increase your fibre intake and stay well hydrated by drinking at least 2 litres of water a day – more in hot weather or if you are exercising.
- See Self-Help for Constipation (page 10).

Ignoring the Urge to Go

Busy, hectic lifestyles often mean we ignore the sensations that tell us we need to open our bowels. Sometimes embarrassment at asking for the toilet or shyness may play a part. Repeatedly ignoring our body's natural signals increases the chance of chronic constipation developing, as the body gradually becomes less responsive to the normal neuromuscular 'requests' to open the bowels.

Who can it affect? People of all ages.

Incidence: Common.

Age-bias: None.

Symptoms: Constipation.

What can you do?
- Listen to your body and respond when you feel even a faint desire to open your bowels. This should help, although a long-term habit of ignoring your bowels cannot be corrected overnight and will take time.
- Try to establish a habit if you don't have one. Choose the time of day you most often open your bowels, and sit on the toilet (take a newspaper if you like). Don't strain or force anything and don't stay longer than a few minutes, because this will only cause problems (like encourage haemorrhoids). You may find that after a few tries, it starts to work.
- See Self-Help for Constipation (page 10).

Taking Antibiotics

Many common antibiotics – like amoxicillin, ciprofloxacin, erythromycin and tetracycline – list diarrhoea as a common side effect. However, it is generally mild and self-limiting. (Diarrhoea can occasionally be severe. This can be the result of a condition called pseudomembranous colitis, which is caused by the bacterium *Clostridium difficile* becoming overpopulated within the gut, as a result of taking the antibiotics that kill off other gut flora.)

Who can this affect? Anyone who has recently taken antibiotics.

Incidence: Fairly common.

Age-bias: None.

Risk factors: None known.

Symptoms: Diarrhoea.

What can your doctor do?
- If you suspect your diarrhoea may be linked with antibiotic treatment, tell your doctor. He may be able to prescribe an alternative drug. However, never stop taking prescribed antibiotics except on medical advice.
- If diarrhoea is severe, or persists for more than 2–3 days in adults (24 hours in babies, infants and the elderly or frail), seek medical advice.

What can you do?
- Drink plenty of fluids.
- Take a probiotic supplement containing *Lactobacillus acidophilus*, *Bifidobacterium longum*, and *B. bifidum* to restore a good balance of gut flora.
- See Self-Help for Diarrhoea (page 14).

Further Information:
For pseudomembranous colitis, see The Merck Manual,
www.merck.com/pubs/mmanual/section3/chapter29/29a.htm

(Over)use of Aspirin

Although aspirin (acetylsalicylic acid) is one of the world's most popular drugs, it can cause gastric irritation and sometimes bleeding. Aspirin not only thins the blood, but irritates the sensitive membranes lining the stomach and upper small intestine. It can also cause bleeding or ulcers if taken over prolonged periods or in large quantities.

Who can this affect? Anyone using aspirin.

Incidence: Considering that aspirin is used by millions of people every day, problems with it are not unduly common. About six per cent of aspirin users report gastric upsets.

Age-bias: None known (children under the age of 12 should never be given aspirin, as it can trigger a rare but serious condition called Reye's Syndrome).

Risk factors:
- A susceptibility to ulcers (if you have ulcers you may be warned off aspirin altogether).
- A history of digestive problems.
- Smoking.
- A tendency to stress.

Symptoms:
- Gnawing or burning feelings in the stomach and chest, similar to heartburn, can signal gastric irritation.
- Dark, almost black, stools can indicate bleeding from the stomach or small intestine.
- If the bleeding has been going on for a long time, you may feel tired and look pale and anaemic.

Always seek medical help urgently if you have severe bleeding or suddenly develop additional symptoms like faintness, dizziness, shortness of breath, pallor and abdominal pain.

What can you do?

- Except for low doses given to prevent blood clotting, never use aspirin for more than two days without your doctor's or pharmacist's advice.
- Liquorice or peppermint tea can help soothe the stomach and mucous membranes. Marshmallow root, comfrey and slippery elm may also help.
- Antacids may relieve any irritation caused by aspirin use.
- See Self-Help for Bleeding (page 20).

Prescription and Non-prescription Drugs

Some drugs like fluoxetine (Prozac) and some non-steroidal anti-inflammatory drugs for pain relief – like indomethacin, and mefenamic acid (e.g. Ponstan) – can cause diarrhoea. Others, including certain tranquillizers and some other kinds of antidepressants, can cause constipation. Painkillers and cough medicines that contain codeine, antacids containing aluminium or calcium, and multivitamins containing iron may also cause constipation, although some people find that iron tablets give them diarrhoea.

Who can they affect? Anyone prescribed these drugs, or taking over-the-counter medicines or supplements.

Incidence: Relatively uncommon.

Age-bias: None.

Risk factors: None known.

Symptoms: Diarrhoea or constipation.

What can your doctor or pharmacist do?

- Check with your pharmacist if you suspect your problem may be caused by your medication.

Do not stop taking any prescribed or recommended medication unless a medical professional has specifically advised you to.

What can you do?

■ See Self-Help for Diarrhoea (page 14) or Constipation (page 10).

CHAPTER 6

How Diet and Nutritional Problems Affect the Digestive System

It is accepted fact that diet can affect many aspects of physical health. The food we eat plays a vital role in virtually every process in the body – providing energy, enabling the body to grow, fighting off disease, repairing tissue and so on – and if we don't provide the body with what it needs, it will be unable to carry out these tasks to the best of its ability.

Unfortunately, the media are full of scare stories giving us regular doses of conflicting advice about what we should or shouldn't be eating. One minute it's bad for you, the next, it isn't. However, look behind the headlines and you'll find that the advice is the same as ever: try to eat a varied diet that largely consists of unprocessed foods. That means plenty of fruit and vegetables; a range of high quality protein sources such as fresh fish, chicken and pulses; unrefined carbohydrates such as brown rice, wholemeal bread and brown pasta; and limit the amount of saturated fat you eat in favour of healthier sources of fat such as olive and fish oils. Whilst I would not claim that a good diet is a panacea for gut problems, remember that it provides your body with the tools to fight infection and ill health so it is a vital part of a holistic approach.

Increasingly, functional foods are also being seen as an important component of a good diet and probiotics in particular are an important step forward in good gut health (we discuss this in greater detail on page 247).

In this chapter we look at the way diet can affect the digestive system – how too little or too much of certain foods may cause gut problems – and how food intolerances and allergies affect gut health.

Chronic Dehydration

Long-term, or chronic, dehydration is a common problem and one that affects not just our gut, but also our energy levels. We need to drink around 2 litres (about 8 glasses) of water (or fluids) every day, but many people constantly drink less than this amount.

Who can it affect? Anyone – although very busy people are most prone as they sometimes ignore thirst or drink too many diuretic drinks like coffee, tea and caffeinated soft drinks.

Incidence: Incredibly common. The Natural Mineral Water Information Service estimates that 90 per cent of people in the UK don't drink enough water to stay healthy and well hydrated.

Age-bias: Chronic dehydration can affect people of any age.

Symptoms:
- Constipation
- Thirst
- Infrequent urination
- Dark, strong–smelling urine
- Lethargy

What can you do?
- Increase your fluid intake to 2 litres a day. This amount does not include caffeinated drinks or alcohol – if you drink a lot of these you will need to drink even more water to counter their diuretic effect.
- Make it a habit to sip constantly from a glass of water at your desk, in the kitchen, from a bottle in the car, or wherever you spend most of your time.
- Avoid drinking too much liquid in the evening otherwise you will be woken at night with a full bladder. Instead, drink more, earlier in the day.
- See Self–Help for Constipation (page 10).

If you constantly feel very thirsty, need to wee a lot, feel unduly tired or lethargic, see your doctor; this can be a sign of diabetes.

Are You Dehydrated?

Answer the following questions to see if you're dehydrated...

- Does your mouth feel dry? If it does, you're already dehydrated.
- Do you feel thirsty? If you do, you're also already dehydrated.
- What colour is your urine? Strong-smelling, dark urine is a sign of dehydration. Urine should be pale straw coloured.
- Are you moody? Dehydration can cause mood swings.
- Pinch the skin on the back of your hand. Does it bounce back quickly? If not, it may be another sign of dehydration. (Think of plants – their leaves also become floppy if they're not well watered.)
- How many glasses of liquid do you drink a day? If it's fewer than eight, you're probably dehydrated – especially if you drink caffeinated drinks, which are diuretic and can increase your body's water loss.
- Do you get frequent headaches? This is often a sign of dehydration – so before you reach for the aspirins, have a couple of glasses of water first.
- Does your facial skin feel dry and need frequent moisturizing? Most of the moisture our skin gets comes from within. Your beauty regime will be much more successful if you are well hydrated.

Caffeine

The *Journal of Internal Medicine* recently described a woman who suffered chronic wasting, vomiting and diarrhoea. Her symptoms turned out to be caused by caffeine poisoning – she had been drinking *8 litres* of caffeinated drinks *every day* over several years, giving her about 1g of caffeine daily. Obviously, most people aren't this excessive. However, caffeine is a powerful stimulant that exerts unwanted effects on our bodies if we take too much – or more than we're used to.

Who can it affect? Anyone who drinks caffeinated drinks – teas, coffee, cola and 'energy' drinks like Red Bull – or anyone taking caffeine tablets.

Incidence: Relatively common.

Age-bias: None, although students and young adults often take caffeine as a stimulant to keep them awake for long periods of study, work or for late-night partying.

Risk factors: Some people are more sensitive to caffeine than others. Caffeine may also exaggerate the effects of alcohol.

Symptoms of excess caffeine:

- Diarrhoea
- Headaches (which can also happen after withdrawal from caffeine)
- Tremors
- Palpitations
- Sleeplessness
- Restlessness
- Anxiety
- Sweating

What can you do?

- Limit yourself to three or four caffeinated drinks a day. Remember that caffeine is found in many drinks – tea, colas, high-energy drinks, chocolate and other products.
- See Self-Help for Diarrhoea (page 14).

Further Information:
Norfolk Mental Health Care NHS Trust Pharmacy Medicine Information
Web Site, www.nmhct.nhs.uk/pharmacy/caff.htm
University Health Services, University of California, Berkeley,
www.uhs.berkeley.edu/HealthInfo/EdHandouts/caffeine.htm

Fibre

Fibre is hugely important to gut health on many levels. If your body lacks fibre, food waste passes through the gut very slowly. The muscular intestines need physical bulk to squeeze against, to push waste along. Hard, impacted faeces not only cause constipation, but can lead to the development of haemorrhoids and anal fissures. They also predispose people to developing diverticular disease in later life, where the bowel walls are stretched and develop weak spots (pouches) that are prone to infection. Stools that progress slowly through the bowel allow toxins and carcinogenic substances to be in contact with bowel wall cells for lengthy periods. This may be one factor that influences the development of colorectal cancers. Conversely, a diet high in fibre contributes to a regular and healthy bowel habit, promotes the presence of healthy gut bacteria, prevents constipation and lowers the chances of developing a whole range of bowel and anal problems.

Fibre binds to and helps lower cholesterol, and slows down glucose absorption into the bloodstream, thereby helping to regulate blood sugar levels. Fibre also absorbs any excess oestrogen that our bodies try to dispose of – a lack of dietary fibre can lead to this waste oestrogen being reabsorbed. Prolonged exposure to oestrogen and certain oestrogen-mimicking chemicals (xenoestrogens) has been linked with the development of many cancers, most notably those affecting the reproductive organs.

So fibre is great – but in the right quantity. Although constipation due to lack of fibre is extremely common, the answer is not to suddenly start eating large amounts of fibrous food. A sudden and large increase in your fibre intake can cause wind, bloating, abdominal pain and diarrhoea (especially in children). The key is to always increase your fibre intake gradually.

Who can fibre-related problems affect? Anyone.

Incidence: Fibre-related gut problems (most notably constipation) are incredibly common in the developed world, and less so in developing countries. Diarrhoea and wind because of a sudden increase in fibre intake are also common among people who are trying a new, healthy diet regime.

Age-bias: None.

Risk factors: Highly processed, high fat and high sugar diets are notoriously low in fibre.

Symptoms:

■ Too little fibre can cause constipation and abdominal discomfort.

■ Too much fibre can cause diarrhoea, wind, bloating and stomach discomfort.

What can you do?

■ If you think eating too little fibre causes your constipation, start by adding some bran cereal or dried fruit to your diet for a few days, drink more water, and see what happens.

■ Always introduce fibre gradually. If it causes problems (like diarrhoea or wind) reduce the amount, keeping it at a level your body is comfortable with for a week or two. Then start *gradually* increasing it again.

■ See Self–Help for Constipation (page 10), Diarrhoea (page 14), and Wind and Bloating (page 27).

Strongly Coloured Foods and 'False' Bleeding

'False' bleeding occurs when you have symptoms that suggest you're bleeding from your gut, when in fact you are not. Iron pills can make the stools look black – a sign that can easily be misinterpreted as bleeding from higher up in the gut, while certain foods like beetroot and blueberries can dye your stools red.

Who can this affect? Anyone taking iron supplements (for example, anyone being treated for anaemia), or anyone who has eaten highly coloured foods like beetroot or certain berries.

Incidence: Not uncommon.

Age–bias: None, although women in their reproductive years often take extra iron so are more prone.

Risk factors: None.

Symptoms: None.

What can you do?

- If you have eaten beetroot, blueberries, or other strong-coloured foods, have no other symptoms and feel completely well, any red-coloured bowel movements occurring 24–36 hours afterwards are most likely caused by what you've eaten. If you are still worried, see a doctor urgently as bleeding from the gut can indicate a serious problem.
- Some people find iron pills make them either constipated or give them diarrhoea. If you are taking iron supplements, stop them for a day or two to see if your stools return to a more 'normal' colour. If your doctor has prescribed them, however, do not stop taking them until or unless he advises otherwise. Tell your doctor at your next visit.

Inadequate Nutrition through Malabsorption

Malabsorption happens when the small intestine is unable to absorb some of the nutrients our bodies need. This normally happens as a result of damage to the walls of the small intestine, or because of a lack of certain enzymes that would normally break down foods so that they can be absorbed into the bloodstream.

Who can it affect?

- Malabsorption can affect people with hormone or enzyme disorders – for example, pancreatic disease can prevent the pancreas from producing specific digestive juices, and people with lactose intolerance may lack the enzyme lactase needed to break down milk sugars.
- Crohn's disease, coeliac disease or even infections like Giardiasis can cause damage to the intestinal lining.
- Diabetics are prone to abnormal gut movement and malabsorption because of nerve damage that sometimes happens to the muscles of the small intestine.
- People may also be affected if they have had long segments of small intestine removed – known as 'short bowel syndrome'.

Incidence: Fairly infrequent.

Age-bias: Any age-bias will be related to the specific cause of malabsorption.

Risk factors: Predisposing conditions include

- Chronic pancreatitis
- Cystic fibrosis
- Lactose intolerance – see page 81
- Coeliac disease – see page 85
- Crohn's disease – see page 153
- Giardiasis – see page 112
- Scleroderma, a disease that causes connective tissue to thicken and harden
- Diabetes

Symptoms: While these depend on the underlying illness, they may include

- Bulky, pale and foul-smelling diarrhoea
- Wind and abdominal bloating
- Weight loss
- Abdominal pain
- Tiredness and lethargy
- Anaemia may result if the underlying condition is left untreated

What can your doctor do?

- Proper diagnosis of malabsorption is essential so that treatment for the underlying condition can be given.
- Treating the cause of malabsorption normally resolves the problem.
- Vitamin supplements (possibly including vitamin B12 injections) can be given if necessary.

What can you do?

- See Self-Help for Diarrhoea (page 14), Wind and Bloating (page 27) and Abdominal Pain (page 24).

Further information:

British Diabetic Association, www.diabetes.org.uk

The Coeliac Society, www.coeliac.co.uk

International Foundation for Functional Gastrointestinal Disorders (US), www.iffgd.org

The National Association for Colitis and Crohn's Disease, www.nacc.org.uk

Food Allergy and Intolerance

First let's look at the difference between an allergy and an intolerance. Food allergy causes the immune system to react against a specific protein or molecule, and produces symptoms such as breathing difficulties and hives (urticaria) that can be specifically identified as being caused by a particular food. These symptoms can be serious and sometimes life threatening (see the symptoms list below). The term food intolerance tends to be applied when a particular food makes a person feel unwell with symptoms that do not involve the immune system and are not directly connected with an allergic reaction. These may include symptoms like diarrhoea, migraine and aches and pains. Because of the nature of the symptoms it can be difficult to prove that they are caused by a particular food. Below we look at some of the common and not-so-common allergies and intolerances and some of the latest findings:

- **Egg allergy** An allergy to eggs (normally egg white, the albumen) is more common among children than adults; reactions can be severe. Apart from food, watch out for vaccinations that may have been cultured using eggs.
- **Nut allergies** These are most often linked in people's minds with anaphylactic shock – a severe and life-threatening reaction that as little as 1/44,000th of a peanut can cause. (Peanuts are, in fact, not nuts but legumes. However, they are commonly thought of as nuts and included in discussions about nut allergies.) However, few food allergies, even those to peanuts, are of the severest form (which involve breathing difficulties, swelling of the throat and closure of the airway, a drop in blood pressure and unconsciousness), although anyone who also suffers with asthma, or who has experienced reactions even to a tiny sample of the food allergen, may be more at risk of developing anaphylactic reactions in the future.
- **Fructose** Recent research from the universities of Iowa and Kansas shows that intolerance to fructose, a simple sugar found in honey and many fruits, may explain some of the symptoms of IBS, which typically causes abdominal pain, bloating and constipation or diarrhoea. The studies, involving fructose breath tests of patients with unexplained gastrointestinal problems, found an abnormal presence of hydrogen or methane gas in over 75 per cent of the patients – the presence of these gases indicates that fructose is not being digested normally.

- <u>Histamine</u> This can occur naturally in certain foods (like cheese, some kinds of wine and fish such as tuna and mackerel) and can trigger what appears to be an allergic reaction. In fact it is simply an 'overload' response to high levels of histamine present in food and is called histamine toxicity.

- <u>Food additives</u> Adverse reactions to food additives can occasionally occur – for example, yellow dye number 5 (tartrazine) may occasionally cause hives (a skin rash). Some experts believe that certain additives may cause hyperactivity in susceptible children, although other authorities dispute this.

- <u>Monosodium glutamate</u> (MSG) This flavour enhancer, used in processed foods and sometimes in oriental cuisine, can cause flushing, feelings of warmth, headaches, sinus pressure and chest pain in some people.

- <u>Sulphites</u> These can occur naturally in food, or can be added as a preservative, which, according to the US-based National Institute of Allergy and Infectious Diseases (NIAID), may occasionally cause problems for asthmatics.

- <u>Exercise</u> Some people occasionally develop allergic reactions to certain foods (usually celery or shellfish) if they eat them before undertaking strenuous exercise. This is because exercise makes the body temperature increase and this, combined with eating a trigger food, can induce symptoms similar to classic food allergy. These include itchiness, light-headedness and hives or even anaphylaxis. The same food would not cause symptoms if it were eaten without exercising afterwards.

Who do these problems affect? It's hard to say, as there is a surprising degree of dispute between various authorities about the real figures. Up to 20 per cent of the British population believe they suffer with food intolerance or allergy. However, a report from the British Nutrition Foundation estimates that most of these cases are unproven and that only a small proportion (perhaps 1–2 per cent) of adults are genuinely intolerant of certain foods. The British Allergy Foundation, however, estimates that up to 40 per cent of the UK population 'suffer some kind of adverse reaction to food'.

The NIAID claims that 'only about three per cent of children have clinically proven allergic reactions to foods', although they point out there is a real difference between food *allergy* and food *intolerance*.

Incidence: Numbers are hotly disputed. Between 1 and 2 per cent of the adult population are believed to have a genuine food allergy and up to 40 per cent of people may suffer varying degrees of food intolerance.

Age-bias: Food allergy and intolerance can affect any age and occasionally run in families. Many studies from different countries around the world suggest that food intolerance (especially lactose intolerance) is more common in children, affecting 5–8 per cent of them.

Risk factors:

- **Parents** – If both your parents have allergies, you are more likely to develop them than if you only have one (or no) parent with allergies.
- **Existing allergies** – If you have allergies to other substances (e.g. latex, pollen), you are more likely to have food-related allergies.
- **Weaning** – Some experts believe that weaning infants too early may be linked to food intolerance in later life.
- **Pregnancy** – Eating foods commonly associated with allergies (like peanuts or shellfish) during pregnancy may also increase the risk of food allergies subsequently developing in children.
- **Breast-feeding** – Many experts believe that breast-feeding delays the onset of food allergies in your baby, and may minimize the chances of them happening altogether. Although the jury is still out on this, the 'breast is best' rule is worth following, especially if you have a family history of allergies and intolerances.

Symptoms:

- Abdominal upsets like diarrhoea and stomach aches
- Headaches
- Muscular aches
- Skin reactions – urticaria ('hives'), flushing, eczema
- Swelling of the lips, mouth or throat
- Breathing difficulties
- Vomiting

If symptoms are severe, seek help immediately. They may indicate a serious food allergy that can cause anaphylactic shock. Symptoms of anaphylaxis include:

- Sudden feelings of extreme anxiety
- Swelling of the face, lips and tongue
- Breathing difficulties

- An itchy red rash
- Dizziness
- Loss of consciousness

IF ANY OF THESE HAPPEN, SEEK EMERGENCY MEDICAL TREATMENT

> Occasionally, symptoms similar to those of food intolerance may be caused by food that is contaminated by toxins – for example, from rodent excrement, insects, mould, bacteria, parasites and viruses.

What can your doctor do?
- He will advise you whether your symptoms indicate food intolerance or allergy. Be prepared to answer the following questions:
  - How quickly did the reaction occur after eating the suspected food? Timing is a good indicator of food allergy.
  - How much of the food did you eat? Sometimes allergies are triggered only after eating certain quantities of a food.
  - Do you *always* have this reaction when you eat the suspected food? Allergies can develop 'from nowhere', but once they appear they generally continue consistently.
  - If you've had a bad food reaction, were you the only person that experienced it, or did it affect others who ate the same foods with you? Histamine or food poisoning, for example, will generally affect everyone who eats a contaminated food, not one isolated person.
  - How was the food prepared? Sometimes raw or undercooked fish can cause an allergic reaction, while the same fish cooked properly won't have any effect at all.
  - Are you allergic to any other known substances? Known allergens often cause cross-reactivity with other substances.

What can you do?
- Take preventative measures for your children. 'Friendly' bacteria (probiotics) given to babies during weaning may help alleviate the symptoms of eczema and connected allergies, suggests research in the medical journal *GUT*.

- **Get tested:**
  - If you suspect food allergy or intolerance, you can be tested using a skin patch test. A dilute extract of the food is placed on your forearm or back and then lightly scratched with a needle, using a control area for comparison. If it produces marked swelling or redness, it can indicate sensitivity to the food, although you do get false positive responses with scratch tests.
  - You cannot try skin tests if your allergy is severe enough to cause anaphylaxis. They are also not suitable for anyone with skin problems like severe eczema or psoriasis.
  - Blood tests like the RAST test detect the presence of a food-specific antibody in the blood, but are not always foolproof.
  - The 'gold-standard' for allergy testing is the double-blind food challenge, where various foods, some containing the suspected allergen and some not, are put in opaque capsules. After each one is swallowed, a reaction is watched for. This should only be done in an appropriate medical setting as severe reactions are possible. It is time-consuming and expensive, and not terribly useful if you're trying to pinpoint the cause of multiple allergies.
  - There are a growing number of independent food allergy testing services providing, for example, the IgG food intolerance test, which, despite being clinically unproven (and expensive), is increasing in popularity and – after encouraging anecdotal reports – has been endorsed by the British Allergy Foundation.

  Other popular (although clinically unproven) tests for food allergy include:
  - Cytotoxicity testing, where a suspect food allergen is added to a blood sample, to see if it causes the white blood cells to 'die'.
  - Sublingual (under the tongue) or subcutaneous (under the skin) provocative challenges which introduce the suspected offending food to see if the patient's reported symptoms worsen or not.
- **Eliminate the suspects:**
  - If you suspect you know which food (or food group) upsets you, eliminate it from your diet for *at least* a few days to see if your problems improve.
  - Formal elimination diets can be very restrictive and should only be carried out with the guidance of a qualified nutritionist or medical professional.
  - Some processed foods contain many different ingredients, so be aware of 'hidden' sources of the food you are trying to avoid.

- Keep a food diary, listing what you eat and how you feel each day.
- If fructose intolerance is a possibility, try to eliminate this sugar from your diet – this will mean avoiding fruit, honey and other processed foods which may contain fructose, such as fruit juices and juice drinks, and fruit-flavoured produce. Read food labels carefully – fructose is widely used.

- Don't eat for at least two hours before exercising. Avoid celery and shellfish before exercising, as these are most commonly linked with exercise-induced food allergy.
- Serious allergy sufferers – especially those likely to experience anaphylactic shock – must always be prepared in case they are accidentally exposed to their allergen.
  - Wear a medical bracelet or necklace that states your allergy details.
  - Antihistamines can help relieve cases of hives, sneezing and gastric ill-effects, and bronchodilators can help if the food allergy triggers asthma.
  - Always carry epinephrine if your allergy may cause anaphylactic shock ('Epi-pens', which are self-contained doses of epinephrine with an integral syringe, can be self-administered).
  - Parents of allergic children should always inform their school and other carers about the child's condition – and make sure that they know how to carry out emergency treatment.
  - 'Desensitizing' treatments may sometimes be effective over time.
- See Self-Help for Diarrhoea (page 14) and Abdominal Pain (page 24).

Further information:
The British Allergy Foundation (Allergy UK) – www.allergyfoundation.com
National Institute of Allergy and Infectious Diseases – www.niaid.nih.gov/factsheets/food.htm
British Nutrition Foundation – www.nutrition.org.uk

Cross-Reactivity – What Is It?

If you have an allergy to prawns, your doctor is likely to suggest you avoid all similar shellfish – for instance, crab, lobster, scampi and so on – because the specific allergen in prawns is also likely be found in other related species. This is cross-reactivity and, in this case, is the result of foods being related and therefore chemically alike. However, cross-reactivity works in other ways, too:

for instance, the NIAID says that ragweed sensitivity cross-reacts with several other plants and foods – for example, melons (especially cantaloupes), sunflower seeds, cucumbers and bananas. If you eat them, they may give you intense itching in your mouth ('oral allergy syndrome'). There is also a link between birch pollen allergy and sensitivity to eating apple skins – despite the fact that they are not related. The cause of such cases of cross-reactivity appears to lie in the fact that these plant products – although unrelated – contain the same kind of small molecules, called phenols.

Latex, widely used in condoms, balloons and rubber gloves, is a plant derivative that contains about 240 proteins, of which over 50 are known allergens. People with latex allergy often cross-react to apples, avocado, bananas, chestnuts, cherries and other stone-fruit.

Lactose Intolerance

Lactose intolerance (hypolactasia), often wrongly seen as a food allergy, is actually the result of the small intestine becoming increasingly unable to produce enough lactase, the enzyme needed to digest lactose, the main sugar in milk. Lactase is produced by special cells in the lining of the small intestine. Normally, lactase breaks lactose into two simpler and easily digested sugars – glucose and galactose, which are then absorbed into the bloodstream for use by the body. When there isn't enough lactase to digest all the lactose in the small intestine, the lactose starts to ferment, causing bloating, abdominal discomfort or pain, diarrhoea and sometimes vomiting.

Who can it affect? Certain racial groups are more vulnerable – up to 90 per cent of Asians, 75 per cent of Africans and significant proportions of people from Eastern Europe and the Mediterranean experience some degree of lactose intolerance. The least vulnerable group are people of northern European descent.

Incidence: Lactose intolerance is very common, affecting an estimated 10 per cent of the global population.

Age–bias: Lactose intolerance is only rarely present from birth. It tends to develop over time, as the amount of lactase our bodies produce decreases as we get older. Lactose intolerance is often first noticed in teenagers and young adults (unless it is the temporary kind which may follow a bout of gastroenteritis).

Risk factors:
- Racial origins that may predispose you to lactose intolerance
- Gastroenteritis may cause temporary lactose intolerance if the lining of the small intestine is affected
- Coeliac disease
- Genetic inheritance

Symptoms: (these usually start 30 minutes to 2 hours after eating or drinking lactose-containing foods – normally dairy produce)
- Bloating
- Wind
- Abdominal cramps and pain
- Diarrhoea
- Nausea and vomiting

What can your doctor do?
- Several tests can be done to identify lactose intolerance, although a doctor may be able to diagnose it from your description of your symptoms. Tests include:
  - Giving a dose of milk after fasting and waiting for symptoms.
  - A breath test. This measures the amount of hydrogen in the breath and can indicate that undigested lactose is being fermented by bacteria, resulting in excess hydrogen gas being produced.
  - A biopsy of the small intestines, during which a tiny sample of the gut lining is taken and analysed for the presence of lactase.
  - Blood tests that identify the levels of blood glucose and galactose after lactose has been ingested (after fasting). If blood glucose and galactose levels remain low, it means that the lactose is not being broken down properly, indicating insufficient amounts of lactase enzymes.

■ Stool acidity tests. Undigested lactose that becomes fermented by bacteria leads to the formation of lactic acid that can be detected in stool samples.

What can you do?

■ Avoid lactose. Those who have a *shortage* of lactase enzymes can usually get away with simply avoiding the main sources of lactose. However, if you have an acute sensitivity, which can happen in (rare) cases of genetically inherited lactose deficiency, you will also need to avoid 'hidden' sources of lactose. Hidden sources aren't normally a problem for the average sufferer, as most people can tolerate small amounts of lactose, but those with an acute sensitivity need to be aware of just how much lactose sneaks into everyday food products. Apart from avoiding dairy produce, you may have to watch out for the following, all of which can contain hidden lactose:
  ■ Bread and other baked goods
  ■ Breakfast cereals (muesli often contains dried milk powder)
  ■ Soups
  ■ Breakfast drinks
  ■ Margarine
  ■ Processed meats
  ■ Salad dressings, dips (many contain cream or cheese)
  ■ Various sweets and snacks, especially chocolate and ice creams
  ■ Medicines – 20 per cent of medicines contain lactose in their base formulation
■ Check food labels. Lactose often appears in food labels under the cloak of a different name. The following milk products all contain lactose: casein, caseinate, sodium caseinate, whey, lactoglobulin, lactalbumen, and curds.
■ Supplements: Lactase supplements are available – these can either be added to ordinary milk to 'predigest' up to around 70 per cent of the normal lactose content, or they can be taken orally as capsules. To relieve colic in babies, try 'Colief' Infant Drops, which contain lactase to help break down milk sugars.
■ Look out for lactose-free foods – these are increasingly available in health food stores and larger supermarkets. Brands include:
  ■ Provamel (soya-based desserts and milk)
  ■ Rakusen's (kosher non-dairy spreads and ice-creams)
  ■ Plamil foods (non-dairy 'milk', chocolate bars, mayonnaise and dairy-free desserts), Rice Dream (non-dairy beverage)

83

- The Stamp Collection (Buxton Foods) dairy-free sheep's cheeses
- Vitasoy (soya drink), Soymage (cream cheese alternative) and Vitaquell (non-dairy margarine spread)
- Lactose-reduced products are also increasingly available.
- See Self-Help for Nausea (page 17), Diarrhoea (page 14), Abdominal Pain (page 24), and Wind and Bloating (page 27).

Further information:

National Digestive Diseases Information Clearinghouse – www.niddk.nih.gov/health/digest/pubs/lactose/lactose.htm

The British Allergy Foundation (Allergy UK) – www.allergyfoundation.com

American Dietetic Association – www.eatright.org/

How to Get Enough Calcium on a Dairy-Free Diet

Dairy foods are an important source of calcium, so if you have a dairy-free diet, you must ensure your calcium intake doesn't suffer. The most important reason is to avoid osteoporosis as you age; your bones and teeth rely heavily on calcium to retain their strength. Calcium is also important for muscle development and blood clotting. (Make sure you are also getting adequate amounts of vitamin D, which helps in the absorption of calcium. Exposure to sunlight helps our skins to manufacture vitamin D.) The average adult needs 1,000 mgs of calcium every day, while pregnant or breastfeeding mothers, the elderly and teenagers need 1,300mgs. So how can you get your quota if you're dairy-free? Here are some alternative calcium-rich foods:

- Green vegetables like broccoli, Chinese cabbage, greens, kale and olives
- Dried fruit – figs, apricots, sultanas, currants, pineapple, pears, mixed peel, dates and glace cherries
- Nuts (hazelnuts, almonds, brazil nuts) and nut products (e.g. tahini)
- Small fish that are normally eaten with the bones – choose sardines, anchovies, pilchards, whitebait
- Shellfish like oysters and shrimp
- Molasses, tofu and carob flour

If you are worried about the amount of calcium in your diet, calcium supplements are widely available at pharmacies and health food stores.

Coeliac Disease (Coeliac Sprue, 'Wheat Allergy' or Gluten Sensitivity)

'Looking back, I realize that I suffered with digestive problems for more than 20 years. During my teens, I often had alternating diarrhoea and constipation and a distended stomach, which I put down to raging teenage hormones. I also suffered from migraines, like my mother. After certain meals, I would find myself belching and bloated and unable to go to the loo for a couple of days. I thought it must be normal. Of course, now that I have a healthy gut, I know it wasn't normal at all.

Later, I started experiencing intense stomach pains. Eventually, in desperation, I cut out dairy products. It made no difference; then I tried eliminating wheat. I felt fantastic. Eventually, during a particularly busy period, I went back to my "old" eating habit and, no surprise, the bloated stomach, constipation and general irritable bowel symptoms returned almost immediately. I suspected that I had wheat intolerance and have rarely touched wheat products since. It means no bread, no pasta, no cakes or chocolate, plus a lot of other foods like sauces made with flour.

I do eat well, though   yoghurt and oat biscuits, lots of milk. I eat a lot of salads, vegetables and rice. I don't think that being wheat-free is a hardship, especially as nowadays foods are so clearly labelled, and I am so lucky to have been able to leave behind those debilitating symptoms.'

Dana, 36, who has coeliac disease

Coeliac disease is caused by the body's inability to tolerate gluten, a complex protein found not just in wheat, but also in rye, barley and oats. (Recent Finnish research suggests that oats may not in fact exert any harmful effects but it is too early to draw any firm conclusions). Some coeliacs are supersensitive to gluten and can be made ill by as little as 200 parts per million of gluten. Gluten is made up of two smaller proteins – glutenin and gliadin; in coeliacs, these proteins trigger the immune system to attack the lining of the small intestine. The immune-triggered response leads to flattening of the villi, the tiny finger-like projections that line the small intestine in their millions, and which normally enable nutrients to be absorbed into the bloodstream. Imagine the villi-covered intestinal lining is like shag-pile carpet; with coeliac disease the lining (with its flattened villi) essentially becomes as flat as linoleum. As a result, food passes through the gut without being absorbed properly.

Who can it affect?

- It used to be thought that coeliac disease only affected children. In fact, it affects people of all ages.
- Most people are diagnosed when aged 35–40 years old.

Incidence: Experts now suspect that coeliac disease is much more prevalent than initially thought. As many as one in every 100 people may have gluten intolerance.

Age-bias: None.

Risk factors:

- There seems to be a genetic link in a large percentage of coeliacs, although research suggests that a number of genes (such as the HLA gene) are involved.
- Recent research by the Medical College of Wisconsin also reveals that people with insulin-dependent diabetes may be even more likely to have coeliac disease, although they don't know why.

Symptoms:

- Pale, bulky, foul-smelling stools
- Diarrhoea
- Weight loss (or failure to gain weight in children)
- Nausea and vomiting
- Anaemia
- Fatigue
- Tiredness, occasionally breathlessness
- Abdominal discomfort
- Mouth ulcers

These common symptoms can be acute, mild and chronic – or anywhere in between. Another possible sign of gluten sensitivity is dermatitis herpetiformis, a very itchy skin rash with red, raised patches of skin and small blisters on the elbows, buttocks and knees. Research at the Royal Hallamshire Hospital in Sheffield, UK, has shown that loss of co-ordination may also be caused by gluten sensitivity (known as 'gluten ataxia'). The cerebellum (the part of the brain responsible for coordination) and the neurons that extend out from it are most susceptible to gluten ataxia.

What can your doctor do?

- Because the symptoms of coeliac disease are very similar to certain other medical conditions, coeliac disease can be difficult to diagnose. Doctors can test for endomysial antibodies in the blood (an EMA test). If positive, they would confirm it with an intestinal biopsy (tissue sample), done under mild sedation.
- Left untreated, coeliac disease can cause serious problems:
  - Malnourishment can lead to vitamin and mineral deficiencies, anaemia and osteoporosis.
  - Coeliacs are more prone to some gastrointestinal cancers and suffer more respiratory illnesses.
  - Women with coeliac disease have a higher incidence of infertility and miscarriage, and often give birth to smaller babies.
- If there are worries about osteoporosis, your doctor may suggest a bone density (DEXA) scan to measure the amount of calcium in your bones.

What can you do?

- Basically, stick to a gluten-free diet (see box overleaf). If you do, your body will absorb more of the nutrients, vitamins and minerals it needs to keep you healthy. Staying gluten-free is also vital if you want to avoid developing osteoporosis. There is also a higher incidence of small intestinal malignancies among untreated coeliacs and strict adherence to a gluten-free diet may lower this risk. According to the Primary Care Society for Gastroenterology, the proportion of coeliacs complying with a gluten-free diet may be as low as 45 per cent.
- See Self-Help for Nausea (page 17), Diarrhoea (page 14), and Abdominal Pain (page 24).

Further information:
Coeliac UK patients' support group, Helpline 0870 4448804
www.coeliac.co.uk
The Celiac Disease & Gluten-free Diet Support Page www.celiac.com
Canadian Celiac Association (CCA) www.celiac.ca

www.nowheat.com – a useful personal site with good links through to a wealth of other pages.

Living a Gluten-Free Life

Key Tips

- Use separate cooking and serving utensils from that of the rest of the family to avoid cross-contamination – especially important for supersensitive coeliacs.

- Take minerals or supplements if advised by your doctor – if you're newly diagnosed you may be low in certain nutrients, probably calcium and vitamin D. Be aware, though, that some medicines, vitamins and mineral supplements may contain gluten.

- Eating out can pose a problem. Be direct with your hosts and explain exactly what you can't eat – most people will appreciate being told rather than having to guess.

- Many (but not all) products are well labelled, so do check carefully for hidden gluten – soy sauce, for instance, contains wheat, and 'modified starch' and 'hydrolysed vegetable protein' may (but not always) contain gluten. Coeliac UK produce a very useful Food and Drink Directory listing gluten-free products. E-mail publications@coeliac.co.uk or call 0870 4448804.

- Gluten-free flour, bread, biscuits and pasta are available on prescription.

- Educate your friends and family about your disease and encourage them to support you.

Don't Eat

- Bread, cakes, pastries and biscuits
- Pasta and pizzas
- Processed foods – like sausages, hamburgers, fish fingers, fish cakes, chicken nuggets – that contain breadcrumbs
- Battered products – like fish, Yorkshire puddings, pancakes and crepes
- Wheat cereals and yoghurts that contain muesli or grains
- Malt, rusk, thickeners and modified starches which may contain wheat

- Dried mustard powder, dried stock cubes, soy sauce and certain canned soups
- Processed cheeses and meats, pâtés and instant mashed potatoes, as well as sauces, gravies and some salad dressings
- Semolina, couscous and many puddings and desserts – including sugar strands and some other cake decorations
- Drinks that may contain gluten, such as malted milk and barley water. (Beer, lager and stout are also made from barley and contain gluten.) Also milkshakes – they may include wheat-based thickeners

Do Eat
- Plenty of fruits and vegetables
- Unprocessed fish, meats and cheese
- Wheat substitutes – corn, potato, rice, barley, soy and rice flours, sago and arrowroot starches will make important contributions to your carbohydrate needs. You can use combinations of these to good effect
- Polenta (made with potato flour) – it's a good substitute for pasta
- Dairy produce – yoghurts, milk, fromage frais

CHAPTER 7

How Problems of the Reproductive System Can Affect your Guts

Apart from organs that we all possess – like intestines and bladders – women also have ovaries, wombs, fallopian tubes and so on. By comparison, the male reproductive organs are either located outside the abdomen (e.g. testicles and penis) or are much smaller and less intrusive (like the prostate gland which sits neatly around the urethra like a little doughnut).

During pregnancy there are obviously added pressures on the body – the uterus grows to many times its original size and there's a baby (sometimes more than one) thrashing about. But even when things are relatively quiet, there's still a monthly period with muscular contractions to contend with. It can get even worse when things go wrong – if, for example, an ovarian cyst develops it can occasionally grow to an enormous size, filling the entire abdomen. No wonder it's hard for women to tell whether lower abdominal pain is caused by gut or reproductive problems. Many doctors can't tell either, until there's been at least some investigation. There's just too much going on down there! This chapter looks at the problems of the reproductive system that commonly cause gut-related symptoms. Most of this chapter is relevant just to women, although problems like the STI chlamydia and Toxic Shock Syndrome can also affect men.

Period Pains

The severity of period pains varies widely from one individual to the next – some have a tolerable amount of pain whilst others suffer terribly (abnormally difficult or painful periods is known as dysmenorrhoea). Painful periods are believed to be caused by higher than normal levels of prostaglandin hormones – these are responsible for making the uterus contract so that the (unfertilized) womb lining can be shed each month. To make matters worse, periods can also cause problems such as diarrhoea and constipation.

Incidence: Extremely common.

Who can it affect?

- Anyone having her period, though women taking oral contraceptives report it less often.
- Dysmenorrhoea often runs in families.
- One study reports that period pains are significantly worse in women with a low dietary intake of fish oils (omega-3 fatty acids EPA and DHA).

Age-bias: Painful periods tend to happen earlier in a woman's reproductive life and may improve after having children, but not always.

Risk factors: The following can cause painful periods, or make the pains worse:

- A uterus that tilts backwards instead of forwards (a retroverted uterus)
- Lack of exercise
- Emotional stress
- Endometriosis (a disorder that affects the womb lining)
- A narrow cervical canal
- Fibroids

Symptoms:

- Lower abdominal pain, sometimes radiating to the thighs and lower back
- Constipation or diarrhoea
- Headaches
- Nausea

What can your doctor do?

- In severe cases, your doctor may advise you to take oral contraceptives.
- He may also investigate further if there may be complicating factors like endometriosis.

What can you do?

■ Take painkillers — several brands are specifically designed for tackling period pain like Feminax, Ibufem and Librofem.

■ Vitamins and Supplements: Increase your intake of omega-3 fish oils. Vitamin B6 can also help prevent menstrual cramps, and iron and zinc are useful for heavy bleeding. (Iron is essential for production of red blood cells and zinc is needed to maintain a healthy reproductive system generally.)

■ Herbal help: Evening Primrose oil capsules are excellent for PMS and period pains and peppermint or catnip tea can help relieve abdominal cramps.

■ Aromatherapy: Cypress, clary sage and lavender oils can help ease painful cramps.

■ Ayurvedic medicine: Caraway is useful for relaxing the uterus to relieve cramping pains, while cardamom helps digestive problems associated with periods.

■ Take warm baths or place a hot-water bottle on the abdomen.

■ See Self-Help for Nausea (page 17), Diarrhoea (page 14), Constipation (page 10), and Abdominal Pain (page 24).

Further information:
BUPA,
http://hcd2.bupa.co.uk/fact_sheets/mosby_factsheets/Dysmenorrhoea.html

Constipation during Pregnancy

Constipation in pregnancy is often caused by the growing weight of the uterus putting pressure on the bowel.

Who can it affect? Expectant mothers, especially during the last three months of a pregnancy.

Incidence: Fairly common.

Age-bias: Women of childbearing age.

Symptoms:

- Constipation. Constipation will also increase the chance of developing haemorrhoids, a condition common during pregnancy.

What can your doctor do?

- Your midwife or doctor can advise on the best way to relieve constipation.

Pregnant women must always be cautious about taking herbal or other supplements – some of them may have unwanted or even dangerous effects on a pregnancy.

What can you do?

- Always tell your doctor or midwife if constipation persists for more than 2 weeks.
- Dietary help:
  - Gradually increase your fibre intake.
  - Drink more fluids – in addition, a glass of tepid water with a slice of fresh lemon before breakfast often helps move things along.
  - Fybogel and bulking agents made from ispaghula husk can also help, especially if you are finding it hard to eat enough fibre because of nausea or food cravings.
- Herbal help: Fennel and ginger act as gentle laxatives and are safe for preventing constipation.
- Ayurvedic medicine: Eating caraway seeds can help relieve constipation, as can mustard (either powdered or seeds).
- Aromatherapy: A combination of geranium, fennel, marjoram and ylang-ylang oils used in a bath is reported to help constipation.
- See Self-Help for Constipation (page 10).

Further information:
Make Way for Baby, www.makewayforbaby.com/prenatalcare.htm

An Important Note about Pregnancy

It is especially important during pregnancy that any unusual pains, sensations, or events are always mentioned to a doctor. Certain conditions like miscarriage, placental abruption (where the placenta comes away from the womb lining) and even ectopic pregnancies can cause abdominal pains, bleeding and so on, and you should seek medical help at the earliest opportunity if you are, or suspect you could be, pregnant.

ALWAYS ASSUME THAT ANY PROBLEM MAY BE CONNECTED WITH YOUR PREGNANCY, UNTIL OR UNLESS YOUR DOCTOR REASSURES YOU THAT IT ISN'T.

Chlamydia

Chlamydia is probably the most common sexually transmitted infection today. It is known as a 'silent epidemic' because 75 per cent of women and 50 per cent of men who have the infection have no symptoms. However, when it does cause symptoms, these can be confused with gut problems. Because it can lead to pelvic inflammatory disease (PID) in women or an infection inside the testicles (called epidydimitis) in men if left untreated, it has the potential to affect the fertility of vast numbers of people in later years.

Who can it affect? Sexually active men and women.

Incidence: With 4 million new cases in the US every year, it has become the most widespread STI (particularly among under-25s).

Age-bias: None, although it is especially prevalent among teens and young adults.

Risk factors:
- Unprotected vaginal or anal sex
- Multiple partners

Symptoms:

The majority of infected people show no symptoms. When present, they include

- Abnormal discharge from the vagina or penis.
- Pain on urinating.
- Chlamydia can inflame the lining of the rectum, and also cause 'pink eye'.
- Women may experience low abdominal pain, painful intercourse and bleeding between periods.

What can your doctor do?

- If you are infected, have both yourself and your partner treated, avoiding sex until the infection is fully cleared.
- Antibiotics like azithromycin and doxycycline are generally used with good results.

What can you do?

- Protect yourself by using condoms during sex.
- If you have had a course of antibiotics, follow it with probiotics like *L. acidophilus, B. longum* and *B. bifidum* to repopulate your gut with good bacteria.
- Herbal help: Fresh garlic and Echinacea both act as immune system stimulators to help the body fight infections.
- Vitamin boosters: Vitamins C, E and the mineral zinc help tissue healing and recovery and boost the immune system.
- See Self-Help for Abdominal Pain (page 24).

Further information:

AfraidToAsk.com, www.afraidtoask.com/STD/index.html (Note: this site contains some explicit pictures)

NetDoctor, www.netdoctor.co.uk/diseases/facts/chlamydia.htm

Endometriosis

Doctors are uncertain about why the tissue which normally lines the uterus occasionally starts to grow in other places – like on the ovaries, in the fallopian tubes, the lower intestines or pelvic cavity. This tissue, the endometrium, thickens during the course of a normal menstrual cycle in preparation for pregnancy and, when a woman doesn't become pregnant, the endometrium is then shed (this is what makes a period). Misplaced endometrial tissue still responds to the female hormones that trigger menstruation, but instead bleeds into the pelvic cavity or fallopian tubes, causing irritation and considerable discomfort.

Who can it affect? Because endometriosis is intrinsically linked with the menstrual cycle, it can only affect women and girls with active reproductive systems.

Incidence: Endometriosis is estimated to affect up to one in every five women.

Age-bias: Girls and women aged between approximately 11 and 48.

Risk factors: Women in their 30s who have not had any children are more likely to develop endometriosis.

Symptoms:
- Pain in lower abdomen (normally felt just before and during periods)
- Irregular or heavy periods
- Painful sex
- Painful urination
- Diarrhoea or constipation

What can your doctor do? There are several treatments for endometriosis:
- Combined oral contraceptives (containing oestrogen and progesterone) may be given.
- Hormone therapy (using various synthetic hormones) can prevent menstruation.
- Lasers can be used during laparascopic procedures to destroy small pieces of endometrial tissue, although they can grow back again.
- Removal of the uterus and ovaries is a last resort for the severest cases.

What can you do?

- Chinese herbal medicine: Da Huang (Rhubarb) is sometimes used to treat 'stagnant blood' complaints like endometriosis.
- Homeopathy: Aconite can help relieve the sharp pains endometriosis can cause.
- Vitamin boosters: Vitamins A and E help maintain healthy reproductive tissue.
- See Self-Help for Diarrhoea (page 14), Constipation (page 10), and Abdominal Pain (page 24).

Further information:

The National Endometriosis Society, www.endo.org.uk/info.html
Endometriosis.org, www.endometriosis.org/

Ovarian Cysts

There are several types of ovarian cyst, which are quite common in women of reproductive age. Most are harmless, cause no symptoms and disappear without any need for treatment. Generally, the size of the cyst rather than the type indicates whether or not there is pain and other symptoms. Large cysts (which can grow to the size of a grapefruit or larger) interfere with organs like the bowel, which may result in symptoms similar to irritable bowel, including diarrhoea and constipation, feelings of fullness and bloating, and pain. Some cysts can indicate ovarian cancer, but this is rare. In such cases, there would normally be additional symptoms such as abdominal swelling, persistent nausea or heartburn, appetite loss and pelvic pain.

The list below covers the main types of ovarian cyst:

- Functional cysts are quite common and develop in the normal course of ovulation. They normally disappear within a few months, causing minor or no symptoms.
- Dermoid cysts are (bizarrely) formed of various kinds of body tissues – hair, fat, skin, even teeth – and are mostly small and cause no symptoms.
- Cystadenomas develop from cells on the outside of the ovary and can grow very large, causing pain and interfering with other abdominal organs.
- Endometriomas are cysts formed from endometrial tissue that has migrated from the uterus (see Endometriosis, above). Because they regularly fill with

blood, they are red/brown in appearance and can be painful during a menstrual period.

- Multiple cysts often form with a condition called Polycystic Ovary Syndrome (PCOS), which causes irregular periods, weight gain, acne, facial and body hair, and infertility.

Who can they affect? Cysts can affect any woman, particularly in her reproductive years when the ovaries are active.

Incidence: Ovarian cysts are an extremely common gynaecological problem, with functional cysts being the most prevalent. Polycystic ovarian cysts affect 4–7 per cent of women.

Age–bias: Women in their fertile years.

Risk factors: None known.

Symptoms:
Depending on the type and size of cyst these can include:
- Abdominal pain
- Painful intercourse
- PCOS additionally causes increased body hair, weight gain, irregular periods and infertility

What can your doctor do?
- Always seek medical advice if you suspect you have a cyst. The majority of functional cysts disappear slowly over a few weeks, although you may need a few ultrasound scans to check the cyst's progress.
- Treatments, depending on the type and size of cyst, range from simple hormone treatment to surgery.

What can you do?
- Don't panic: The majority of ovarian cysts are harmless and disappear on their own within a few months.

- Herbal help:
  - Vitex agnus castus (also known as 'chaste tree' and 'monk's pepper') may help balance oestrogen levels.
  - Blue cohosh is typically used for conditions affecting the reproductive organs, although it should not be taken by anyone with angina, and can irritate gastrointestinal symptoms. It should always be avoided during pregnancy.
- Aromatherapy: Clary sage can help balance hormones, and lavender, neroli, jasmine and vetivert all have anti-anxiety properties.
- Vitamin boosters: Vitamin E can help in the prevention and treatment of cysts and B-complex can help with hormone balance.
- See Self-Help for Abdominal Pain (page 24).

Further information:
The Mayo Clinic, www.mayoclinic.com/invoke.cfm?id=DS00129
The Polycystic Ovaries Self Help Group, www.verity-pcos.org.uk/

Ovarian Cancer

Ovarian cancer is one of the most common cancers among women in the UK. Scientists have yet to pinpoint the cause of ovarian cancer, although there do appear to be both hormonal and genetic factors involved. Ovarian tumours sometimes develop from ovarian cysts.

Who can it affect? Women during and after their reproductive years.

Incidence: Around 7,000 women are diagnosed with ovarian cancer each year in the UK, making it the 4th most common female cancer (after breast, bowel and lung cancer). The UK has among the highest incidence of ovarian cancer in Europe.

Age-bias: Ovarian cancer can affect relatively young women, although the typical age for developing it is over 45. The chances of developing it increase with age – it is most commonly diagnosed in women aged between 65 and 74.

Risk factors:
- If a close relative has suffered from ovarian cancer under the age of 50, your chances of developing it also may be slightly increased.
- Women who have never had children may be more at risk.
- Women who have entered the menopause later than average may also be marginally more at risk.
- Diets high in animal fat are believed to contribute to the risk of developing ovarian cancer.
- Some doctors believe that intimate use of talcum powder may also increase the risks of ovarian cancer developing, if the powder travels up into the woman's body and irritates cells.
- There is also some evidence that fertility treatment may marginally increase your risk of developing this type of cancer.

Symptoms: One of the biggest problems with diagnosing ovarian cancer is that during the early stages of the disease, there are often few or no noticeable symptoms. When they do appear, they may include:
- Lower abdominal pain
- An unusual change in the bowel habit (unexplained constipation or diarrhoea)
- Swelling in the abdomen (from fluid)
- Occasional vaginal bleeding
- A frequent desire to pass urine
- General symptoms of cancer – like weight loss, nausea and vomiting

These symptoms can be misdiagnosed as irritable bowel syndrome, so if there is a history of ovarian cancer (or bowel cancer) in your family, mention this and ask for screening.

What can your doctor do?
- Surgery to remove the ovaries and uterus (womb) is an almost inevitable part of treatment in all but the earliest stages of the disease.
- Chemotherapy is given, using the drugs carboplatin or cisplatin and possibly also paclitaxel (Taxol).
- Radiotherapy is another treatment option that normally follows surgery.

What can you do?

- Some experts suggest that having children while you are young – and breastfeeding them – may reduce your risk of ovarian cancer.
- Doctors are fairly sure that using the combined (oestrogen and progesterone) pill does confer some degree of protection against ovarian cancer.
- Avoid a diet high in saturated (animal) fats.
- Avoid using talcum powder intimately.
- See Self-Help for Nausea (page 17), Diarrhoea (page 14), Constipation (page 10), and Abdominal Pain (page 24).

Further information:

National Ovarian Cancer Coalition www.ovarian.org

Cancer Research UK, www.cancerhelp.org.uk/help/default.asp?page=143

Toxic Shock Syndrome (TSS)

TSS occurs when a bacterial poison invades the bloodstream. The poison is produced by the bacterium *Staphylococcus aureus* (and also by some *streptococcal* bacteria).

Who can it affect?

- About half of all cases of TSS occur in women having their periods. The condition has been linked to tampons, which can provide an ideal breeding ground for these bacteria, especially if left in situ for extended periods of time or 'lost' in the vagina.
- TSS can also affect anyone exposed to these bacteria through an infected wound.

Incidence: TSS is extremely rare. There are fewer than about two dozen reported cases of TSS in the UK every year (in a population exceeding 58 million).

Age-bias: Most common in women aged between 15 and 20.

Risk factors: Using tampons for extended periods of time may be a risk factor.

Symptoms:

- Sudden onset of fever
- Vomiting
- Diarrhoea
- Muscle aches and pains
- A sunburn-like rash may also appear over the body

What can your doctor do?

- Once identified, TSS is generally easily treated using antibiotics and intravenous (IV) fluids to increase the patient's blood pressure.
- You may be advised to permanently stop using tampons, as TSS can recur.

What can you do?

- Always keep cuts and wounds clean (and covered if necessary) to prevent infection from setting in or spreading.
- Avoid using tampons for long periods of time, particularly overnight.
- Use the lowest absorbency tampon that you can, and alternate with towels.
- Always insert tampons with clean hands to avoid introducing bacteria.
- Never use more than one tampon inside the vagina.

Further information:

Toxic Shock Syndrome Information Service, www.toxicshock.com

CHAPTER 8

The Thyroid and its Effect on the Digestive System

The body operates as a *system* and with any system there is always overlap between the various component parts as they function together. This means that certain problems that arise outside the gut may sometimes inadvertently affect it. An especially good example is the thyroid gland, which is discussed in this section. This gland, located in the front of the throat, produces hormones that affect the way our body metabolizes (uses) energy. You'd be excused for thinking that it has no obvious link to the digestive system – but it does. When the thyroid gland goes into overdrive, it tends to cause nervous and jittery symptoms. One of them (and often one of the first) includes diarrhoea. Conversely, when the thyroid is acting too sluggish, it may cause us to suffer with constipation.

Underactive Thyroid (Hypothyroidism or Myxoedema)

The butterfly-shaped thyroid gland – which sits at the base of the throat around the trachea (windpipe) – produces hormones that have important influences over many aspects of our body's metabolism, especially energy use. A 'sleepy' or underactive thyroid gland fails to produce enough thyroid hormones, which causes many body functions to slow down. Constipation is a common side effect.

A common cause of hypothyroidism is infection (thyroiditis), which can itself be caused by an autoimmune disorder (Hashimoto's thyroiditis), a viral infection or can occur as a consequence of pregnancy. Hashimoto's disease is an autoimmune disorder in which antibodies are produced that attack the thyroid gland, causing permanent damage to the organ. Hashimoto's tends to run in families. With viral infection and post-partum thyroiditis, the resulting hypothyroidism is usually temporary. Viral and post-partum thyroiditis typically cause overactivity (hyperthyroidism) of the thyroid, followed by underactivity (hypothyroidism).

Thyroid problems are sometimes associated with other diseases, such as pernicious anaemia, diabetes or rheumatoid arthritis. An underactive thyroid may occasionally follow trauma or surgery. Inadequate intake of dietary iodine – which is vital for the production of thyroid hormones – can also cause underactivity. Very rarely, an underactive thyroid can be caused by pituitary problems.

Who can it affect? Thyroid problems generally affect women more than men and may run in families. Researchers believe there may be a link with the female hormones.

Incidence: About 1 in every 100 people.

Age-bias: Usually in the 40 plus age-range, though it can occur earlier. It is most common in the over-65s. As many as 1 in 10 women over the age of 65 may be showing signs of hypothyroidism, according to the American Thyroid Association.

Risk factors:
■ A diet lacking in iodine
■ Hashimoto's disease

Symptoms:
■ Extreme tiredness
■ Constipation
■ Weight gain
■ Hoarseness of the voice
■ Feeling excessively cold
■ Puffiness of the face (especially around the eyes)
■ Dry, thickened skin
■ Hair loss
■ Heavy periods (in women)
■ Swelling of the neck (called a goitre)

What can your doctor do?

- Always see your doctor if you suspect you have an underactive thyroid. It usually requires treatment (which may vary depending on the cause) and monitoring.
- A blood test can be done to measure the amount of thyroid hormones present and detect antibodies that attack the thyroid gland.
- Synthetic thyroid hormone (thyroxine) is commonly prescribed for underactive thyroid problems. Symptoms generally start improving within about 3 weeks. (If the problem is caused by inflammation of the gland – i.e. viral thyroiditis or post-pregnancy thyroiditis – the situation will often rectify itself spontaneously.)
- Regular monitoring with blood tests ensures the correct dosage is being given.

What can you do?

- Herbal help: Bladderwrack may help regulate thyroid function and reduce any goitre.
- Aromatherapy: Geranium oil in a bath or in massage oil is beneficial for balancing hormones, as is clary sage.
- Dietary help: Food sources of iodine are important – an underactive thyroid gland can sometimes result from a dietary deficiency. Eat plenty of onions, garlic, salt (iodized), bread, dairy produce and fish. It's also important to make sure you're not deficient in zinc, vitamin A, selenium and iron – found in meat, nuts, pulses, eggs and leafy green vegetables.
- Don't overdo the iodine: Much as dietary iodine is important for the thyroid to function effectively, it is equally important not to take too much. Generally speaking, the amount that occurs naturally in food is non-toxic – but watch out for high-dose supplements. The normal recommended amount is 140 micrograms (mcg) for adults daily; the safe maximum is around 1,000mcg daily. Prolonged use of large amounts of iodine (6,000mcg or more daily) can suppress the thyroid's natural hormone production, which may lead to underactive thyroid problems.
- See Self-Help for Constipation (page 10).

Further information:
The American Thyroid Association,
www.thyroid.org/resources/patients/brochures/hypothyroidism.html
The Thyroid Society, www.the-thyroid-society.org/

Overactive Thyroid (Hyperthyroidism, Graves' Disease)

An overactive thyroid occurs when there is overproduction of thyroid hormones. Seventy-five per cent of all cases of overactive thyroid are due to Graves' disease – which happens when the immune system attacks the thyroid gland, causing it to overproduce thyroid hormones. This speeds up the body's metabolism, causing it to 'run' a lot faster than normal. In the same way that an underactive thyroid leads to constipation, an overactive thyroid can cause diarrhoea.

An overactive thyroid may also be caused by inflammation of the thyroid (thyroiditis) that is triggered by a viral infection or pregnancy. Hyperthyroidism is also occasionally associated with other autoimmune disorders like vitiligo and pernicious anaemia, or as a result of hormone-producing nodules in the thyroid gland.

Who can it affect? All thyroid problems are 7–10 times more common in females than males and sometimes run in families.

Incidence: The annual incidence of hyperthyroidism in the US is about 1 in 1,000 women (it's negligible in men).

Age-bias: Most commonly affects the 20–50 age group.

Risk factors:
- A family history of Graves' disease – this is thought to have a genetic basis and tends to run in families

Symptoms:
- Diarrhoea
- Weight loss (despite an increased appetite and greater food intake)
- Rapid, sometimes irregular heartbeat
- Hand tremors
- Increased sweating and feelings of undue warmth
- Feelings of anxiety and jitteriness
- Insomnia

- Swelling of the neck (goitre)
- Muscular weakness
- Irregular periods in women
- Bulging eyes (a later sign associated with Graves' disease)

If you suspect a thyroid disorder, always see your doctor for diagnostic tests and treatment. You cannot self-manage thyroid problems.

What can your doctor do?

- The feelings of anxiety and 'jitteriness' that accompany overactive thyroid can normally be suppressed using beta-blocker drugs (like propranolol).
- Overactive thyroid due to Graves' disease is normally treated using anti-thyroid drugs like carbimazole (Neo-Mercazole), propylthiouracil (PTU) and methimazole (Tapazole®), which are taken for up to 18 months. The problem often rectifies spontaneously after this.
- Radioactive iodine can be given (in capsules that are swallowed) to partially destroy the thyroid gland, thus lowering the levels of hormone that it produces.
- Surgery to remove some of the thyroid gland is another option.
- After radioactive treatment and therapy, it is sometimes necessary to supplement using thyroxine hormone to prevent underactivity.

What can you do?

- Diarrhoea should only need to be treated short-term – thyroid conditions don't permanently affect the digestive system and diarrhoea will stop once the condition is being controlled.
- Herbal help: Bugleweed, drunk three times a day, can help an overactive thyroid.
- Chinese herbalism: Marine plants and seaweed are often prescribed for hyperthyroidism, which is believed to be caused by 'heat in the liver'.
- Homeopathy: Iodum may be offered if the patient is hyperactive and feels hot. Rock salt (Natrum muriaticum) and belladonna are also used by homeopaths for treating hyperthyroidism.
- See Self-Help for Diarrhoea (page 14).

Further information:
Endocrine Web (US) – www.endocrineweb.com
Thyroid UK – www.thyroiduk.org

CHAPTER 9

Infectious Illnesses of the Digestive Tract

Bacteria, viruses, parasites and worms can all cause infections – and they can all be transferred from person to person. However, although they can be unpleasant in the extreme, infections are generally either self-limiting, or fairly easily cured by using antibiotics or anti-parasitic medication.

There are many preventative measures we can take to avoid these illnesses, many of which result from sloppy hygiene and overconfidence in the food and water offered in some exotic destinations. As well as the more obvious measures we can take (these are discussed on page 235), increasingly strong evidence is emerging that probiotics may play an important role not only in enhancing our immune systems, but in helping prevent infectious gastric illnesses. Soon we may find that taking probiotics becomes just as common-place a part of our holiday health preparations as vaccinations. The role of probiotics is discussed in detail on page 247.

Bacterial Food Poisoning

Several types of bacteria can cause food poisoning. They commonly include *Campylobacter*, *Salmonella*, *Shigella*, *Staphylococci* strains, *Escherichia coli* strains and *Listeria*. Food generally becomes contaminated when it is kept or stored in conditions that encourage bacteria to thrive – warm temperatures make ideal breeding grounds.

Who can it affect? Anyone. However, pregnant mothers or people with compromised immunity are likely to be more seriously affected if they become infected.

Incidence: Common. Around 100,000 cases are logged in the UK each year and up to 2 million people may be affected.

Age-bias: None, though the very young and elderly are more likely to suffer from serious complications.

Risk factors:
- Foreign travel to less developed countries, especially if you are drinking tap water and eating 'street' food
- Eating under unhygienic conditions (i.e. with dirty hands)
- Eating food that has not been properly stored, cooked or refrigerated
- New research from Ohio State University suggests that too much iron in the diet may leave otherwise healthy people more vulnerable to bacterial infections of the small intestine

Symptoms: (there are several types of bacteria that cause food poisoning and each may induce slightly different symptoms)
- Diarrhoea
- Vomiting
- Mild fever
- Abdominal pain or cramping
- Muscle weakness and paralysis can occur with *Clostridium* poisoning
- Flu-like symptoms are a feature of *listeriosis*
- You may have bloodstained diarrhoea (for example, with *salmonella* or *campylobacter* poisoning)

You should seek medical advice urgently if you have bloodstained diarrhoea or if the problem persists for more than 24–36 hours (less in the elderly or infants).

What can your doctor do?
- Anti-emetic (anti-sickness) drugs may be given to stop vomiting. Other medicines may be given to ease diarrhoea.

- Stool samples may also be taken to try and identify the bacteria responsible.
- Food poisoning can lead to severe dehydration, which, if untreated, may require urgent hospital management using intravenous fluids. The very young, elderly and immune-compromised are more vulnerable.

What can you do?
- Rest.
- Keep your fluid intake up.
- Take rehydration salts to restore your body's chemical balance or make your own: mix 250ml (9fl oz) water or fruit juice with a teaspoon of sugar and a pinch of salt.
- Diet tips:
  - Manuka honey dissolved in warm water can help, as it is a natural antibiotic and anti-inflammatory agent.
  - Suck ice cubes if you cannot keep sips of water down.
  - Live yoghurt or probiotic supplements can help repopulate your gut with friendly bacteria as you recover.
- Herbal help: Slippery elm tea may help ease symptoms.
- See Self-Help for Diarrhoea (page 14), Nausea (page 17), Abdominal Pain (page 24), and Bleeding (page 20).

Further information:
Medical Advisory Service for Travellers Abroad,
www.masta.org/staying/index.html
Centers for Disease Control and Prevention (US),
www.cdc.gov/travel/foodwater.htm

Viral Gastroenteritis

Viral gastroenteritis is generally short-lived and self-limiting. Viruses that typically cause it include:

- Rotavirus or astrovirus, which commonly affects children during winter months, causing mild to severe diarrhoea
- Norwalk virus, which tends to affect older children and adults

Many people develop immunity to these viruses after they have been exposed.

Who can it affect? Anyone. Children are especially susceptible to rotavirus and astrovirus. Babies and the elderly are more at risk of being severely affected.

Incidence: Very common in the western world.

Age-bias: None known.

Risk factors:
- Anyone with immune system deficiencies like AIDS
- People whose immunity is compromised through illness or medication

Symptoms:
- Diarrhoea
- Stomach cramps
- Nausea and/or vomiting
- Mild fever
- Headache
- Sweating and/or chills

Always see your doctor urgently if symptoms persist, if there is a marked deterioration in your condition, if there is severe pain or if bleeding occurs.

What can your doctor do?

Viral infections don't respond to antibiotic treatment. Doctors generally know when a viral 'bug' is doing the rounds, and will not offer antibiotics if they suspect your problem is being caused by a virus.

- Your doctor will suggest you take rehydration salts like Dioralyte or Rehidrat, especially when children, infants and the elderly are affected. If you haven't any in the house, mix 250ml (9fl oz) cooled, boiled water or fruit juice with a teaspoon of sugar and a pinch of salt.
- In severe cases, drugs like metoclopramide (e.g. Maxolon) may be given to help reduce or stop vomiting.
- Hospital admission for IV fluids may occasionally be necessary.

What can you do?
- Dietary tips:
  - Ripe bananas can relieve feelings of nausea and may help thicken your bowel output if you have severe diarrhoea.
  - Honey mixed with warm water can also soothe the digestive tract. Manuka honey from New Zealand is claimed to have anti-inflammatory properties.
- Herbal help: Arrowroot and slippery elm teas are often used to settle the stomach and bowel.
- See Self-Help for Diarrhoea (page 14), Nausea (page 17), and Abdominal Pain (page 24).

Further Information:

The Merck Manual, www.merck.com/pubs/mmanual/section3/chapter28/28f.htm

Protozoan Parasitic Infections: Giardiasis, Amoebiasis (Amoebic Dysentery) and Cryptosporidiosis

These infectious illnesses are caused by microscopically-small protozoan parasites and are passed on by contact with infected faeces either directly, or through contaminated food.

Who can they affect?
- These infections are most common in developing countries where sanitation and water quality are poor.
- Outbreaks do occur in developed countries – for example *Giardia lambia* can be caught in mountainous areas in the US; campers and backpackers in such areas are generally advised never to drink untreated stream water.

Incidence: These infections are more common than you might think – *Giardia lambia*, for example, affects almost 20 per cent of the world's population. Amoebiasis affects about 500 million people worldwide.

Age-bias: They tend to affect infants more than adults.

Risk factors: People with weak or impaired immune systems are more at risk.

Symptoms:

- Symptoms of Giardiasis – explosive, foul-smelling and watery diarrhoea; excessive wind; bloating; weight loss; abdominal pain; nausea and tiredness; loss of appetite and occasionally fever and vomiting.
- Symptoms of Amoebiasis – often none, or there may be mild and intermittent bouts of diarrhoea and abdominal pain.
- Symptoms of Cryptosporidiosis – sometimes none, but can include watery diarrhoea, abdominal pain, fever, nausea and vomiting.

What can your doctor do?

- Parasitic infection can be tricky to diagnose as the symptoms are similar to many other gastrointestinal diseases. In addition, many doctors are unfamiliar with illnesses of this kind. It may be necessary to collect stool samples over several weeks to identify the parasite.
- New tests that can detect the body's immune response are now available and are useful for screening children.
- Parasitic infestation can be treated successfully using antiprotozoal drugs like metronidazole (Flagyl), tinidazole, mepacrine hydrochloride and pyrimethamine (Daraprim). Most are given orally, but some are injected to treat severe infection.

What can you do?

- Prevention is better then cure – follow advice given to travellers about avoiding parasitic and other infections (see box overleaf).
- See Self-Help for Nausea (page 17), Diarrhoea (page 14), Abdominal Pain (page 24), and Wind and Bloating (page 27).

Further information:
Anti-Parasite.com, www.anti-parasite.com/index.html

Traveller's Tips: Preventing Parasitic and Bacterial Infections

- Never drink untreated water in areas where parasitic or bacterial infections are endemic – always avoid tap water and don't even use it to brush your teeth.
- Only drink bottled water that you have opened yourself and avoid ice cubes, which may have been made using tap water.
- Street sellers are occasionally unscrupulous, selling 'pirated' bottled water. Stick to known brands with intact seals.
- Fizzy (canned or bottled) drinks are normally safe. Open them yourself.
- Disinfectants like iodine and water purifying tablets are normally very effective, although not necessarily if the water looks cloudy. Iodine resin water purifiers filter and purify fresh water from all sources.
- Be scrupulous about washing your hands before eating and after going to the bathroom.
- Don't accept 'street food' or eat where the hygiene is suspect.
- Avoid undercooked or raw meat, fish or shellfish.
- Avoid unpasteurized dairy foods.
- Avoid eating salads and always peel fruit or vegetables that are eaten raw.
- Don't assume that because something smells and tastes good, it is safe.

Further information: Medical Advisory Services for Travellers Abroad (MASTA), www.masta.org.uk

Parasitic Worm Infestations

Parasitic worm infestations are caused by several species of worm whose life cycle includes a portion of time living inside the human body. The intestinal roundworm *Ascaris lumbricoides* is most common in tropical and sub-tropical areas and is passed via infected food or drink, due to poor sanitation and the use of human waste as a fertilizer. Schistosomiasis (also called bilharzia) is caused by several species of flatworm called flukes, which affect people who bathe in fresh water lakes, canals, or unchlorinated freshwater pools that contain infested freshwater snails.

There are also three types of large tapeworm that typically infect humans and these are associated with eating undercooked pork, beef or fish that is itself infested. Pork and beef tapeworm infestations occur mostly in developing countries and thorough cooking kills the tapeworm larvae. Fish can be infected with the tapeworm, *Diphyllobothrium latum*, though this is more of a problem in countries where uncooked fish dishes are popular, for example Finland and Japan.

Who can they affect?
- Ascariasis is common in underdeveloped countries, but is very rare in developed countries like the UK, Western Europe, US and Australia.
- Schistosomiasis mostly occurs in developing countries.
- The increasing popularity of raw fish dishes – especially in Scandinavia, Eastern Europe and Japan – does increase the risk of contracting a fish tapeworm.

Incidence: Ascariasis affects a quarter of the world's population at one time or another and schistosomiasis affects 200 million people worldwide. Figures for infection by the fish tapeworm *diphyllobothrium* are unavailable – probably because so many cases go unreported or undiagnosed.

Age-bias: Children tend to be more susceptible to parasitic worm infestations than adults.

Risk factors:
- Foreign travel to less developed destinations
- Eating raw or undercooked food
- Bathing in untreated fresh water

Symptoms:
- Symptoms of ascariasis include diarrhoea and abdominal pain. Worm larvae in the lungs may cause wheezing and coughing and large infestations in the intestines may cause appendicitis or a blockage.
- Symptoms of schistosomiasis include diarrhoea, fever, muscle pains, coughing and vomiting, frequent urination with a burning sensation, and blood in the urine. Untreated infestations can eventually cause colorectal or bladder cancer.

- Symptoms of tapeworms include diarrhoea, mild abdominal pain, increased appetite (with beef and pork tapeworms) and occasionally the sensation of worm segments wriggling out of your back passage. Fish tapeworms occasionally cause megaloblastic anaemia.

What can your doctor do?

- Parasitic worm infestations can be diagnosed with blood, urine or faecal samples.
- Treatment usually depends on the specific worm infestation, but is usually a simple course of oral anthelmintic (anti-worm) medication like mebendazole, albendazole or ivermectin.
- Some anthelmintic drugs (like albendazole) may compromise liver function and their use must be monitored carefully.

What can you do?

- Follow traveller's advice (see earlier box on preventing parasitic infections)
- Dietary tips: Raw garlic is said to be toxic to worms and parasites.
- Herbal help: A mixture of cayenne pepper and senna can be effective in expelling worms.
- Homeopathy: China (a remedy made from Peruvian bark, which also produces quinine) is sometimes used to relieve weakness caused by gastric disturbances.
- See Self-Help for Diarrhoea (page 14), Nausea (page 17), and Abdominal Pain (page 24).

Further information:
Centers for Disease Control and Prevention (US),
www.dpd.cdc.gov/dpdx/HTML/Para_Health.htm
Anti-parasite.com www.anti-parasite.com/index/html

Tropical Worm Infestations

The various tropical worm infestations have a variety of causes. Not all of them cause gut-related symptoms, but the ones discussed here can. Trichinosis comes from eating undercooked pork that contains the cysts of the tiny *Trichinella* worm. Strongyloidiasis is usually caught by walking barefoot on soil contaminated with the *Strongyloides stercoralis* worm.

Whipworm is often caught by children who have accidentally ingested the eggs of the worm *Trichuris trichuria*.

Who can they affect? Tropical worm infestations are virtually only ever seen in patients who have travelled to or lived in the tropics.

Incidence: Very rare in developed countries, fairly common in undeveloped areas.

Age-bias: Children are more prone to infestation than adults, because they play outside in soil and often put dirty hands in their mouths.

Risk factors:
- Foreign travel to undeveloped regions
- Eating undercooked or raw pork
- Walking barefoot in contaminated regions

Symptoms:
- In severe cases, trichinosis causes diarrhoea, vomiting, abdominal and muscular pain and fever. Rarely, it can lead to acute heart failure or an illness similar to meningitis.
- Severe infestation of strongyloides can cause abdominal pain and intermittent periods of constipation and weight loss, but symptoms can also be absent for years if the immune system is strong.
- Trichuriasis causes, in severe cases, bloody diarrhoea, abdominal pain and weight loss.

If you have any of these symptoms and you have been travelling to foreign regions, ensure that you tell your doctor where you have been.

What can your doctor do?
- Blood, tissue or faecal samples will usually confirm a diagnosis.
- Treatment involves giving an appropriate anthelmintic (anti-worm) drug.

What can you do?
- Follow traveller's advice (see earlier box on preventing parasitic infections)

- Avoid eating undercooked or raw food in tropical areas where worm infestations are endemic.
- Use appropriate closed footwear when walking through rural areas.
- See Self-Help for Nausea (page 17), Diarrhoea (page 14), Constipation (page 10), Abdominal Pain (page 24), and Bleeding (page 20).

Further information:
Centers for Disease Control and Prevention,
www.dpd.cdc.gov/dpdx/HTML/Para_Health.htm
Anti-parasite.com, www.anti-parasite.com/index.html

Botulinum Poisoning

Botulism poisoning is a very rare but serious illness caused by the *Clostridium botulinum* bacterium. Adults usually contract it by eating contaminated food or through an infected wound. Very occasionally, it is also contracted by infants who have eaten bacterial spores which then grow in the intestines and release the deadly toxin.

Who can it affect? Anyone.

Incidence: It affects fewer than 100 people in the US every year.

Age-bias: None, although infant botulism poisoning, the most common kind, is contracted only by babies and young infants.

Risk factors:
- Eating (especially) home-canned produce, or food from cans that have been dented, punctured or split, or that have bulging lids.
- Feeding honey to infants under 1 year old, as honey occasionally contains spores of the *botulinum* bacterium.
- Drug users, especially those using black tar heroin, are at greater risk of wound botulism.

Symptoms:

- Initial symptoms (which start anywhere between 6 hours and 10 days after contamination) normally include nausea, constipation, a dry mouth, double or blurred vision and muscle weakness.
- Babies show signs of lethargy, poor feeding, floppy muscle tone and have a weak cry.

What can your doctor do?

- Because botulism is rare and has symptoms similar to Guillain-Barré syndrome or myasthenia gravis, diagnosis can be tricky. Stool and blood serum samples may show the toxin's presence.
- You must tell your doctor if you have used any suspect food products. If possible keep a sample of the food (but not where someone else may eat it).
- Immediate treatment using antitoxin drugs is vital; mechanical ventilation may be necessary if breathing has been affected through muscle paralysis. Ninety per cent of people recover if treated promptly.

What can you do?

- Avoid feeding honey to infants under 1 year old.
- Never eat food from cans that are dented, bulging or split.

Further information:

The Wonderful World of Diseases website (www.diseaseworld.com/) has some good links to botulism factsheets.

Typhoid/Paratyphoid

These infections are actually caused by two strains of the salmonella bacteria – *Salmonella typhi* and *S. paratyphi*. Paratyphoid is generally milder than typhoid.

Infection occurs as a result of ingesting food or water that has been contaminated by unwashed hands – generally in areas with poor sanitation and hygiene.

Who can it affect? Anyone.

Incidence: Typhoid fever is still common in the developing world, affecting roughly 12^1/$_2$ million people every year. In developed countries it is very rare. Most of the 400 cases that occur in the US each year are believed to be caught while travelling.

Age-bias: None known.

Risk factors: Travel to developing countries without vaccination cover.

Symptoms:
- Headache and high fever
- Dry cough
- Abdominal pain
- Constipation, normally followed by diarrhoea
- A rash of spots on the chest, abdomen and back

What can your doctor do?
- Vaccination (by injection or oral dose) is advisable for anyone travelling to a developing country.
- The infections can be treated with antibiotics.
- Serious complications (like intestinal bleeding) can be avoided by early diagnosis.

What can you do?
- Get vaccinated before travelling.
- Practice good hygiene – wash hands thoroughly and avoiding undercooked or raw food and tap water, especially in places where hygiene is suspect. Follow the advice given in Traveller's Tips (see page 114).
- Be aware that some people can become 'silent carriers' of the disease – transmitting the infection to others even though they appear perfectly well. You should therefore exercise caution and not assume someone is 'safe' simply because they appear to be healthy.
- See Self-Help for Diarrhoea (page 14), Constipation (page 10), and Abdominal Pain (page 24).

Further information:
World Water Day 2001, www.worldwaterday.org/disease/typhoid.html

Cholera

The bacterium *Vibrio cholerae* has been historically responsible for millions of deaths and is strongly associated with poor sanitation and hygiene, especially in undeveloped nations.

Who can it affect? Anyone visiting or living in an area where cholera occurs.

Incidence: Cholera is very rare in developed nations. It generally occurs in developing nations – and is often associated with the aftermath of natural disasters like earthquakes.

Age-bias: None known.

Risk factors: Travel to undeveloped areas with poor sanitation.

Symptoms:
■ Vomiting
■ Profuse diarrhoea that resembles 'rice water'

What can your doctor do?
■ Unfortunately, cholera vaccinations are not considered particularly effective.
■ Diagnosis can be confirmed using faecal samples.
■ Hospital treatment is normally needed urgently, to replace lost fluids and minerals intravenously.
■ Antibiotics will also be given.

What can you do?
■ Your best bet for prevention is to observe careful hygiene.
■ Avoid drinking unbottled water, ice cubes in drinks and uncooked food, especially from street stalls.
■ Wash your hands before eating.
■ Avoid raw vegetables and salads, and peel fruit before eating.
■ See Self-Help for Nausea (page 17), Diarrhoea (page 14) and Traveller's Tips (page 114).

Further information:

National Center for Infectious Diseases, www.cdc.gov/travel/cholera.htm

World Health Organisation,
http://www.who.int/emc/diseases/cholera/factstravellers.html

CHAPTER 10

Adhesions and Hernias

Adhesions and hernias share one fundamental feature – they are both caused by physical (anatomical) changes inside the abdominal cavity. Adhesions occur when strands of fibrous tissue form connections between organs or areas inside the abdomen that aren't normally joined together. They usually happen as a result of surgery, although they can be caused by other problems, like endometriosis. Hernias, on the other hand, are caused by weaknesses in the muscles of the abdominal cavity, which allow the intestines, for example, to protrude through. While they too can occur after surgery, a more common cause of hernias is either muscular weakness that develops with age, or straining and lifting heavy objects.

Adhesions

Adhesions are strands of fibrous tissue that form as a part of the healing process after injury, trauma or surgery.

What causes them?
As damaged tissues heal, fibrous strands reconnect them. The problem with adhesions occurs when these fibrous bands occasionally form between organs or body tissues that are not normally connected. Adhesions might cause scar tissue to form around nerves, trapping them, or may simply form in a way and place that creates internal discomfort.

While common, adhesions are less well recognized than they might be, according to the UK Adhesion Society. They say that patients often suffer debilitating side effects and may be mistakenly labelled by doctors as psychological or psychiatric cases. Many sufferers complain that there remains a surprising reluctance to acknowledge the problems that adhesions can cause, and feel unsupported (or disbelieved) by their physician.

Who can they affect?
- Anyone undergoing surgery may develop adhesions, but they can also be caused by:
  - Physical injury or trauma
  - Infections
  - Endometriosis
  - Chemotherapy
  - Radiation
  - Cancer
  - or anything that causes scar tissue to form

Incidence: The UK Adhesion Society estimates that at least 55 per cent of people undergoing surgery develop adhesions, although people are often unaware of any problems as a direct result of them.

Age-bias: None known.

Risk factors:
- Numerous surgical procedures and/or physical injuries.
- Women are more likely to complain of adhesions. This is probably because the pelvic organs, (especially the uterus, ovaries and fallopian tubes) seem more prone to developing adhesions. It is also likely that the abundance of surgery that can happen in this area of a woman's body (e.g. caesareans, hysterectomies, infertility treatments, ovarian cystectomies and so on) all increase the chances of adhesions developing.

Symptoms: Many people with adhesions find they cause no symptoms. However, adhesions may cause:
- Painful intercourse
- Infertility
- Severe pelvic or abdominal pain
- Bowel adhesions may cause twisting or kinking of the bowel, which can in rare cases lead to intestinal obstruction (see page 183).

What can your doctor do?

- According to Dr Stuart Gould, Consultant Physician and Gastroenterologist at Epsom General Hospital in Surrey, 'the problem with adhesions is diagnosing them. There are no simple tests to identify adhesions, or to rule them out. If pain is due to intestinal blockage, imaging methods such as CT or barium studies are occasionally useful if carried out during an acute attack. Laparoscopy is another way to diagnose adhesions but can be risky as the laparoscope (a 'scope inserted through the abdominal wall under a general anaesthetic), may perforate intestine that is stuck to the inside of the abdominal wall by an adhesion.'
- Adhesion 'barriers' are constantly being improved for surgical use: these provide a physical barrier (that normally breaks down over time) between tissues in order to minimize the development of adhesions after surgery.
- Further surgery may be needed to rectify obstructions or the pain caused by adhesions.

What can you do?

- Vitamin boosters: Some sufferers say that antioxidant supplements are useful – they may reduce inflammation. MSM (methylsulphonylmethane) reportedly accelerates wound healing.
- Aromatherapy: Lavender oil is calming and can help ease abdominal pain and heal wounds.
- Herbal help: Peppermint oil acts as an antispasmodic and can help relax bowel muscles. Some treatments for IBS (like Colpermin) can help.
- Use self-help groups – they are a valuable source of information and support.
- See Self-Help for Abdominal Pain (page 24).

Further information:
International Adhesions Society – www.adhesions.org/
The UK Adhesion Society – www.adhesions.org.uk

Hernias

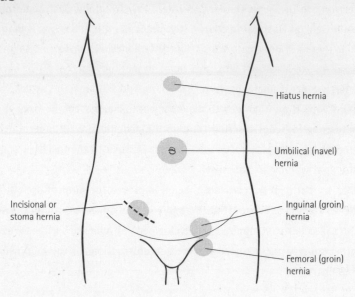

Hernias occur when a part of the intestine or stomach pushes through a weak spot in the abdominal muscles. Hernias can affect the upper or lower abdomen.

What causes them?

- Straining causes a part of the intestine or stomach to protrude through the weak spot. Straining can result from lifting heavy objects, coughing, trying to pass a constipated stool, or simply with increasing age.

- A hiatus hernia happens when the top of the stomach pushes up through the diaphragm, whereas inguinal or femoral hernias occur in the lower abdomen near the groin, when weakened muscles allow the intestine to protrude.

- Umbilical hernias happen in babies, and also when pregnancy stretches the abdominal muscles, and incisional hernias can occur after, for example, a Caesarean section.

- A stoma (an artificial opening on the abdomen where the intestine is brought out onto the surface so that gut waste can be expelled) can create a muscle weakness that later develops into a hernia.

Who can they affect?

- Babies are prone to umbilical hernias, which develop behind the navel – around 1 in 5 babies have an umbilical hernia. Between 3–5 per cent of all newborns will develop an inguinal (or groin) hernia; they are more likely in premature babies.
- Most other types of hernia tend to affect adults – women who have had several pregnancies, men who do heavy lifting or are middle aged, and the elderly.
- Stoma hernias affect people with an ileostomy, a colostomy or a urostomy (an opening from the bladder that drains urine out of the body).
- Hernias are very common – about 1 in 10 of us will have one at some stage.

Age-bias: More common in and after middle age, but this depends on the cause.

Risk factors:
- Being overweight
- Lifting heavy objects
- Being premature (for paediatric hernias)
- Having a stoma

Symptoms:
- A lump in the abdomen or groin which may disappear when you lie down, and which may appear on straining (although not all hernias cause bulges)
- An aching or dragging feeling in the abdomen (although not all hernias cause discomfort)

What can you do?
- Always see your doctor if you suspect a hernia. Occasionally they will twist or strangulate, which may impair the blood supply to the intestine. This is a serious problem that causes severe pain (and possibly vomiting), and warrants immediate surgery.
- Support belts can help prevent undue pressure being exerted on a hernia. They are especially useful for stoma patients.
- If appropriate, lose weight – hernias are more of a problem and more likely to develop if you are overweight.

- Learn to lift properly – it will not only protect you from developing a hernia, but will also spare your back.
- Don't lift more than you can. Being brave doesn't help. Ask for help at supermarkets and when heavy lifting is involved.
- Mothers with young children should bend down to cuddle their children, rather than lifting them up to hold them.

What can your doctor do?

- Doctors can advise if surgery is necessary or if it would help.
- Most adult hernias gradually worsen until they need surgery. However, the outcome is successful in the majority of cases. See Chapter 18, Hospitals, Surgery and More ...
- Paediatric hernias should always be treated as a matter of importance. Umbilical hernias generally close spontaneously, without any need for surgery, although there is a tiny risk that a hernia will become strangulated and require immediate surgery.
- Surgery doesn't always help stoma hernias, especially when they are small and appear to cause no problems. Wearing a wide, supportive ileostomy or colostomy belt can help.

Further information:
The British Hernia Centre, www.hernia.org
Medbroadcast.com,
www.medbroadcast.com/health_topics/health_conditions/hernia/index.shtml

CHAPTER 11

Pains in the Butt – Haemorrhoids, Fissures and Others

For every one case of a serious gut disease, there are dozens of cases of something simple and easily treated – like haemorrhoids. Of course, they can still be intensely painful and troublesome on occasions – and embarrassing, too...

Haemorrhoids (Piles)

Haemorrhoids, commonly known as 'piles', form when veins in the soft tissue around the anus and inside the rectum become swollen. 'External' haemorrhoids form in the outer anal area, while 'internal' haemorrhoids are those located inside the body, in the inner section of the anus and the rectum. Sometimes internal piles may protrude out of the anus; these are called 'prolapsed' or 'prolapsing' haemorrhoids. Piles never turn into cancer.

What causes them?
- Constipation is a key cause of piles: straining to pass a hard stool can lead to excessive pressure on the blood vessels in the rectum, which makes them form swollen piles.
- Usually, piles are not terribly painful, unless they develop clots (thromboses), which can become very inflamed. However, people often fear that opening their bowels will cause piles to hurt and this fear can worsen constipation.
- In pregnancy, the growing weight of the baby can also put pressure on the blood vessels in the rectum, causing piles.

Who can they affect?

- Piles affect at least one third, and possibly as much as half, of the world's population at some point in their lives. Although it's a very common nuisance, it's also a temporary one for many people.
- They are also more common in women during pregnancy and after childbirth.

Age-bias: More common in adults.

Risk factors:

- Constipation
- Straining to pass a stool
- A low-fibre diet
- Being overweight
- Pregnancy
- A job or lifestyle that involves standing a lot

Symptoms:

- Constipation
- Bleeding (bright red), which shows on the toilet paper after a bowel movement
- Mucus discharge
- Itching
- Soreness around the anus
- Sometimes a feeling of incomplete evacuation after opening the bowels
- Occasionally a pile can be felt or seen protruding from the anus

What can your doctor do?

- Various preparatory pile creams (Anusol, Preparation H) can help alleviate pain and itching.
- Topical (i.e. applied locally) corticosteroids may be prescribed for very painful cases.
- Laxatives or stool softeners can help you to pass stools without pain.
- Depending on the severity or location of your piles, your doctor may advise any of the following:
  - Sclerotherapy – This technique involves injecting the pile with a special liquid that makes it shrink.

- Banding – This involves cutting off the blood supply to the pile by placing a small elastic band around the pile; eventually it shrivels up and drops off.
- Persistent piles may be treated surgically (haemorrhoidectomy), and is successful in the vast majority of cases. A new technique using stapling has been developed which is less uncomfortable, although long-term results of the technique are not yet known.

What can you do?

- Always consult your doctor if you are bleeding.
- Avoid straining to pass a bowel motion.
- Increase your intake of fibre – preventing constipation will lower the chances of developing piles. Good foods to eat include prunes, figs, kiwi fruit, spinach, dried apricots, bran and whole grains.
- Bulking agents and stool softeners can be very useful – like psyllium (Metamucil) or methylcellulose (Citrucel – US).
- Practise squeezing your pelvic floor muscles (especially important for pregnant women and anyone who stands a lot). It may not prevent piles from forming, but regular muscular contractions (20–30 a day) will improve the movement of blood in the area and prevent it 'pooling' in veins, which can lead to piles. It will also improve muscle tone and strength, which can help with protruding piles.
- Losing weight will lower your chances of developing piles.
- Herbal help:
  - Witch hazel compresses can help reduce swelling and promote healing.
  - Ointment made from the aptly-named herb pilewort can help.
- Keep the area scrupulously clean: sitting on a bidet and using cold water several times a day can help reduce inflammation. Always pat dry gently using a soft, clean towel.
- See Self-Help for Constipation (page 10), Bleeding (page 20), Mucus (page 21), Itchy Bottom (page 31), and Urgency, Frequency and Incomplete Evacuation (page 29).

Further Information:
The Piles Advisory Bureau,
www.pilesadvice.co.uk

Pruritus Ani

'Pruritus ani' means 'itchy bum'– it's that simple. It affects the anus and the skin immediately surrounding it, and is a surprisingly common problem for adults as well as children.

What causes it? There are many possible causes for this annoying condition. They include the following:

- Antibiotic use. Many broad-spectrum antibiotics (like tetracycline) kill all the good bacteria (as well as the bad ones) and leave the body open to colonization, which results in problems like yeast infections (also called thrush or candida). Thrush can cause itching.
- Skin conditions that leave the skin chronically dry, like psoriasis and atopic dermatitis. Dry skin can be very itchy.
- Excessive sweating.
- Poor hygiene and scratching the skin.
- Irritants like perfumes, washing powders or scented toilet paper can cause irritation or allergic reactions.
- Some foods cause irritation when they are passed in faecal waste. These include chocolate, caffeine, beer, nuts, dairy products, vitamin C and spices.
- Parasitic worm infestations such as pinworm (threadworm) typically cause night-time itching. So can (less commonly) scabies or lice.
- General diseases can often cause skin problems – including diabetes, jaundice and lymphoma (although this is very rare).
- Infections like fungi, bacteria and genital warts can cause itching.
- Itching is a common symptom of piles and may also be associated with problems that cause specific anal lesions like fissures and fistulas.
- Very rarely, cancer may be a cause.

Who can it affect? Anyone, although it tends to happen more to men than women.

Risk factors: Depends on the cause – see the section above.

Symptoms:

- Itching – typically at night or after opening the bowels
- Soreness of the skin around the anal margin, occasionally weeping
- Sometimes a rash in the area

What can your doctor do?

- If there is an obvious underlying cause, the doctor will be able to identify it with a detailed symptom description, physical examination and possibly cultures to identify any infection.
- Doctors can prescribe creams if it is caused by a yeast infection, and can treat threadworm easily with an anthelmintic drug like mebendazole, piperazine (Expelix) or pyrantel.
- Warts or haemorrhoids can be treated successfully with minor surgery.

What can you do?

- Identify the cause. Is it something you ate, or wore? Is it related to exercise or excessive sweating? Think carefully and try to discover the most likely cause.
- Eliminate potential irritants: use plain, soft toilet paper; avoid using scented soap, shower gels or perfumes; wear loose, cotton underwear and avoid nylon pantyhose.
- Use a bidet. Wash after every bowel movement or when itchy and pat dry gently using a soft, clean towel. Avoid rubbing the area.
- Avoid food irritants. Cut out the curries and beer for a while, eat fairly high-fibre food and don't try anything new until you know what causes it.
- If your child has the problem take them to see your doctor – it could be threadworm or an infection that needs attention.
- If you feel unwell, have a fever, are bleeding, can feel a lump or there is a persistent rash, you may need medical treatment.
- See Self-Help for Itchy Bottom (page 31).

Further Information:

St Mark's Hospital advice sheet, www.bowelcontrol.org.uk/pdf/pruritus.pdf

Anal Abscesses

Anal abscesses are pockets of infection that fill with pus. They can be intensely painful. They are normally located close to the anus, but occasionally are located higher up in the anal canal. People occasionally confuse anal abscesses with pilonidal abscesses: pilonidal abscesses are caused by ingrowing hairs in the upper buttock region, and typically affect young, hairy white men.

What causes them? An anal abscess is generally an isolated problem and is not caused by any other underlying illness. It occurs spontaneously when bacteria or a contaminant gets into one of the glands in the anus, where infection develops.

Who can they affect? Men are affected more than women.

Age-bias: More than half of all anal abscesses occur in adults aged between 20–40.

Risk factors:
- Any activity that introduces bacteria to the anal area
- Poor hygiene
- Certain skin conditions (like diabetes), poor immunity and Crohn's disease

Symptoms:
- A firm but tender swelling or lump – sometimes it may be quite large and 'deform' the shape of the anus
- Throbbing pain near the anus, often worse on walking or straining
- Fever, chills and generally feeling unwell or 'fluey'
- Occasionally, pain in the lower abdomen, if the abscess is high up in the anal canal

What can your doctor do?
- A simple physical examination normally reveals an abscess, unless it is located deep inside the anus.

- You may need to have an anoscopy – which involves inserting a small tube into the anus to enable the doctor to see inside.
- Anal abscesses are normally drained surgically, with antibiotics given to treat infection. This procedure is simple and normally done on a day-case or short admission basis.
- Your doctor may want to re-examine you at a later stage, as anal abscesses can result in fistulas (see below).

What can you do?

- Always keep the area clean – this will help prevent any further infection.
- Always use a condom if you have anal intercourse.
- Avoid anal intercourse while an abscess is present or healing.
- See Self-Help for Pain in the Back Passage (page 25).

Further Information:
American Society of Colon & Rectal Surgeons,
www.fascrs.org/brochures/anal-abscess.html

Anal Fistulas

Fistulas happen when an abscess erupts in two directions, making a narrow, tunnel-like passage between two areas of the body that are not normally connected. It's a little like two separate areas of your house being connected by a mouse-tunnel.

Anal fistulas normally form between an existing or previous abscess and the skin surface nearby. Occasionally (in people who have had reconstructive surgery to remove diseased bowel or correct a digestive tract illness), a fistula can occur between, for example, the intestine and the vagina, or between the intestine and the abdominal cavity.

Often, the opening of the fistula on the skin surface leaks a thick, smelly, pus-like substance, which is a result of the abscess still draining contents out of the body. The opening of the fistula can also become blocked up and may cause the old abscess to flare up again.

What causes it? Doctors don't know exactly why fistulas occur, although they are thought to originate mostly from anal gland infections.

Who can it affect? Anyone.

Age-bias: Young adults seem to be more often affected.

Risk factors:
- Anal abscesses
- Prior abdominal reconstructive surgery

Symptoms:
- Pain and discomfort around the anus, normally around the site of an old abscess
- Blood, pus, or unpleasant-smelling mucus oozing from the anal area
- Other symptoms of an anal abscess (see page 134), which would recur if the fistula were blocked and the old abscess 'reactivated'
- If the fistula is between, for example, the intestine and the vagina, intestinal contents may leak into the vagina and be discharged from there

What can your doctor do?
- Fistulas do not heal spontaneously and always need surgical treatment.
- Surgery is generally highly effective – the procedure is called 'laying open' or fistulotomy, and also involves removing all traces of any old abscess. See Chapter 18, Hospitals, Surgery and More ...
- Antibiotics may be given to mop up any residual infection.

What can you do?
- Seek medical help if an abscess appears to recur, worsens, or if you suspect that a fistula has developed.
- Keep the area clean.
- Wear loose, cotton underwear and change it frequently.
- Avoid all anal intercourse until the problem has been treated.
- See Self-Help for Pain in the Back Passage (page 25), Bleeding (page 20), and Mucus (page 21).

Further Information:
St Mark's Hospital advice sheet, www.stmarkshospital.org.uk/pdf/analfistula.pdf

Anal Fissures

Anal fissures are sore-like splits or cracks in the skin at the anal opening. They can be intensely painful, particularly on opening the bowels, as this is when the skin around the anus becomes stretched.

What causes them?
- They typically occur when straining to pass a large, hard stool. Straining overstretches the skin, resulting in a painful tear, or lesion.
- They may be associated with Crohn's disease and UC.
- Less often, they may occur with chronic diarrhoea, or even certain sexually transmitted infections.
- Most anal fissures are superficial, involving only the surface layers of skin, but they may also penetrate the full thickness of the skin.

Who can they affect? Anal fissures are common problems and can affect anybody.

Age-bias: Anal fissures typically affect teenagers and young adults.

Risk factors:
- Constipation
- Chronic bowel disorders like Crohn's disease, UC or IBS
- Anal intercourse
- Insertion of foreign objects into the anal canal

Symptoms:
- Sharp, intense pain that normally accompanies a bowel movement and which may persist for some time afterwards
- Bleeding – small amounts of bright red blood, also typically occurring after a bowel movement
- Itching around the anus

What can your doctor do?

- Stool softeners can help ease the passage of stools through the anus (especially if constipation is a problem).
- Medicated creams can be useful. Glyceryl trinitrate (GTN at 0.2 per cent strength) ointment, developed at St Mark's Hospital, London, has proved successful in healing fissures in over two-thirds of patients tested. According to the *British Medical Journal*, diltiazem hydrochloride (DTZ) 2 per cent ointment also works as well as GTN, but with fewer side-effects (like headaches). Isosorbide dinitrite (ISDN) cream is also available and effective.
- Surgery may be used to treat chronic fissures and is successful in most cases.

What can you do? Many fissures heal spontaneously with self-help measures.
- Try to avoid constipation. Increase your dietary fibre and take bulking agents if necessary. See Self-Help for Constipation, page 10.
- Bathe the affected area in warm, salty water for 15 minutes twice a day.
- Avoid anal intercourse or loveplay while a fissure is healing and always use a condom once it has healed.
- See Self-Help for Pain in the Back Passage (page 25), Bleeding (page 20), and Itchy Bottom (page 31).

Further Information:
Addenbrooke's NHS Trust FAQ,
www.addenbrookes.org.uk/serv/clin/surg/colorectal/fissure1.html

Rectal Prolapse

A rectal prolapse happens when the internal lining of the rectum drops down and protrudes through the anus.

Who can it affect? Generally the elderly, anyone with weak pelvic floor muscles, or anyone who strains excessively when trying to pass a stool.

Age-bias: Rectal prolapses predominantly affect the elderly. Elderly women are six times more likely to develop them than elderly men. They can occur in children of either sex and are associated with excessive straining during toilet-training.

Risk factors:

- Weak pelvic floor muscles
- Spinal injury, which may affect the pelvic floor muscles
- Constipation or straining

Symptoms:

- You may feel a 'lump' protruding from your anus
- Bleeding
- Mucus from the damaged prolapse
- Faecal incontinence occurs in prolapse in about half of patients

What can your doctor do?

- Your doctor will probably investigate the cause to rule out any underlying disease.
- A physician can often gently push the prolapse back up into place with a gloved finger.
- Preventing constipation can help prevent the problem recurring, so he may recommend a change of diet.
- In children, relieving constipation is normally all that is necessary to prevent further problems.

What can you do?

- In children, a rectal prolapse is often caused by a combination of constipation and the strains (physical and mental) of toilet training. The problem usually ceases as soon as constipation is relieved, and with careful potty training.
- In the elderly it may be a considerable problem and usually requires surgical repair. This can be done either through the abdomen to 'hitch up' the rectum, or through the anus to push the rectum back in.
- Always see your doctor to rule out any underlying conditions that may cause a prolapse, such as colorectal cancer.
- See Self-Help for Bleeding (page 20), Mucus (page 21), Pain in the Back Passage (page 25), and Urgency, Frequency and Incomplete Evacuation (page 29).

Further Information:

Colorectal Surgical Society of Australia,

www.cssa.org.au/patientarticle.asp?ArticleNo=22

CHAPTER 12

Irritable Bowel Syndrome or IBS

This functional bowel disorder is medically defined as 'the association of abdominal discomfort with an alteration in bowel habit for which no cause can be found on routine clinical investigation'. The way in which sufferers describe their symptoms gives us far more insight into the debilitating effects of this widespread problem ...

'For the last few years I've had searing pains across my abdomen, bloating, constipation and diarrhoea, nausea and vomiting, and have even passed out because of the pain. My IBS has stripped me of my femininity. I have no energy, I have little self-esteem and I am not the happy, confident person I once was. You feel devastated and isolated until you find someone with the same problem you can talk to – it is a huge relief to find someone who understands how I feel.'

Annie, 27, who suffers from IBS

Functional – What Do They Mean?

Doctors often refer to IBS as a 'functional' bowel disorder. By 'functional' they mean that it affects the way the bowel functions – although no apparent anatomical disease can be identified when the colon is examined. This is what differentiates IBS from the other diseases mentioned in this book. However, IBS is *so* important and affects *so* many people that I could not write this book without giving IBS its own chapter.

According to the Digestive Disorders Foundation, 'A third of people in Britain have occasional symptoms of IBS, and 1 in 10 have symptoms bad enough to require medical attention.' Other research suggests that nearly a third of all referrals to a gastroenterologist are because of IBS. In the US, sufferers of IBS make $3^1/2$ million doctor's visits, receive over 2 million prescriptions and undergo 35,000 hospitalizations *every year*. IBS is a widespread and crippling problem.

Although a few doctors still dismiss IBS as an inconsequential condition, most are increasingly aware of its significance, not just as a serious cause of absenteeism but also as a troublesome and persistent condition that – while it can be mild and intermittent – is also capable of being debilitating and serious.

A Rose by Any Other Name

IBS has masqueraded under several different names over the last 100 years. (Yes, IBS is *not* a disease of the 21st century.) It has also has been called 'colitis', 'mucous colitis', 'spastic colon' and 'spastic bowel'. Most of these terms are inaccurate and are nowadays being replaced by 'IBS'. Remember not to confuse IBS with IBD – it may only be one letter but there is a big difference in terms of diagnosis, treatment and outlook. IBD is discussed in Chapter 13.

Diagnostic Hurdles

One of the common problems faced by IBS sufferers is getting a diagnosis. Many of the symptoms of IBS are similar to those of various bowel or gynaecological conditions. IBS *can* be diagnosed quickly   sometimes there are 'classic' symptom patterns that are easily spotted by experienced gastroenterologists. But equally, it can sometimes involve a series of tests before other causes are ruled out.

To be told something along the lines of 'Well, we can't figure out what else it is, so we'll call it IBS' can leave a nagging worry in the back of your mind that something's been missed. However, because IBS is so very widespread, the chances are more than likely that if no other cause has been found, this is what the problem really is. And having found a diagnosis, it may also mean an end to endoscopies, stool samples and rectal examinations...

What causes it? No one has yet been able to identify an organic cause for this condition. According to Professor Nick Read, a consultant gastroenterologist, analytical psychotherapist and trustee of the IBS Network, 'IBS is probably caused by emotional stress – the visceral expression of unresolved emotional tension.' While this theory is not universally accepted, it is likely that stress is a trigger.

Research shows that the bowels of IBS sufferers are much more sensitive than normal and therefore react to 'triggers' which would not necessarily affect a so-called 'normal' bowel. Some research even indicates that the quality of sleep may be related to the severity of IBS symptoms the following day, especially if a lack of sleep increases levels of stress hormones like adrenaline.

There are some who believe that infections like gastroenteritis, or possibly even antibiotics, may be responsible for causing IBS in certain people. Recent research in the US has indicated that fructose malabsorption may be responsible for IBS-type symptoms in a significant number of healthy people (see also Food Allergy and Intolerance, page 75).

Who can it affect?
- IBS is extremely common in developed countries. In the US, IBS is the second leading cause of worker absenteeism (surpassed only by the common cold) and affects up to an estimated third of the British population at one time or another.
- It affects men and women equally, although women are more likely to seek medical help for it.

Age–bias: IBS most commonly develops between the ages of 15 and 40, but can occur at any age.

Risk factors:
- IBS sometimes runs in families.
- Stress is thought to (at least) aggravate symptoms in some people.
- Too much or too little dietary fibre, a rich or spicy diet, alcohol, caffeine and smoking may all worsen symptoms.
- Research at the University Hospital of South Manchester has reported that the symptoms of IBS can be significantly worse during a menstrual period.

Symptoms: These vary greatly from person to person, which can make diagnosis difficult. Typical symptoms include:

- Abdominal cramping
- Feelings of 'fullness' or bloating
- Unaccustomed changes in the bowel habit like irregularity or alternating between constipation and (painless) diarrhoea, or a predominance of (painless) diarrhoea and constipation
- Wind
- Nausea
- Feelings of urgency (rushing to go to the toilet)
- Pain in the back passage
- Ineffective straining, or feelings of inadequate emptying of the bowel
- Occasionally, pain on sexual intercourse in some women

Bleeding is never associated with IBS (unless you are also suffering from piles) so if you have any blood loss when you visit the bathroom, seek medical attention as soon as possible.

What can your doctor do?
- Ruling out other causes may be important in diagnosing IBS, although sometimes the pattern of symptoms is so characteristic of IBS that simple tests alone may be more than sufficient to confirm a diagnosis.
- Drugs like loperamide (Imodium) can help if diarrhoea is a problem.
- Antispasmodic drugs like atropine (Lomotil), merbentyl (Diarrest), mebeverine (Colofac) and hyoscine (Buscopan) may be prescribed to help reduce colonic and abdominal cramping, diarrhoea and pain.
- Tricyclic antidepressants are sometimes prescribed because they have a calming effect on the bowel.

What can you do?
- See your doctor. A proper diagnosis is necessary to make sure you are treating the right condition.
- Take a 'symptom diary' when you visit your doctor so that he can get the fullest picture possible of your condition.

- Dietary help:
  - Keep a food diary so that you can see if your IBS is caused or aggravated by certain foods.
  - Exclusion diets may help eliminate troublesome foods.
  - Avoid large, spicy, fried and fatty meals.
  - Slowly increase your fibre if constipation is a problem. However, too much fibre, especially if you have diarrhoea, can make things worse.
  - Reduce caffeine-containing drinks.
  - Vitamin A helps keep the digestive tract healthy. Make sure your diet includes enough.
  - Probiotic supplements help keep a good balance of gut bacteria – take live yoghurt, yoghurt-based probiotic drinks or probiotic supplements daily, especially after a course of antibiotics.
- Stop smoking. The gut responds very strongly to nicotine. Avoiding it is best.
- Take regular exercise. This stimulates the body's natural production of 'feel-good' hormones like endorphins, reduces stress and eases constipation.
- Herbal help:
  - Cynara artichoke extract is highly rated by some IBS sufferers – especially for relieving abdominal pain, mucus, constipation, diarrhoea, nausea and urgency.
  - Slippery elm tea can help soothe the gut, as can aloe vera gels and drinks.
  - Peppermint teas and oils are widely used for their help in easing wind, nausea, indigestion and bloating.
  - Ginger and lemon balm are also widely used for their anti-nausea properties and are used to treat many IBS symptoms.
  - Chamomile tea can help ease colicky spasms and windy bloating, and can lower anxiety and promote relaxation.
- Flower remedies: Rescue Remedy can help relieve stress that may trigger an IBS attack.
- Ayurvedic medicine: Coriander and hollyhock are commonly-used herbs for treating IBS.
- Chinese herbal medicine: Chinese medical practitioners may offer several multi-herb preparations for relieving IBS, although they are typically tailored to each individual.

- Hypnotherapy: Gut-directed hypnotherapy has proved useful for some people in relieving IBS.
- Relaxation techniques, such as breathing exercises, yoga and aromatherapy massage, can help alleviate stress.
- Deal with emotional issues. Professor Read says, 'It is important to understand what life situation may have triggered symptoms and deal with that – symptoms are expressions of unresolved emotional tension.'
- Reflexology: Some IBS sufferers claim that reflexology helps relieve tiredness and stress-related symptoms. Reflexology works on the principle that certain points in the feet are related to various parts of the body, and that stimulation of these points using special massage techniques can help relieve problems in the various related body parts. Recent research at the University of Leeds has, however, found that reflexology does not necessarily help alleviate abdominal pain, constipation/diarrhoea and bloatedness.
- See Self-Help for Abdominal Pain (page 24), Diarrhoea (page 14), Constipation (page 10), Wind and Bloating (page 27), Nausea (page 17), Urgency, Frequency and Incomplete Evacuation (page 29), and Pain in the Back Passage (page 25).

Further Information:
National Digestive Diseases Information Clearinghouse,
www.niddk.nih.gov/health/digest/pubs/irrbowel/irrbowel.htm
The IBS Network, www.ibsnetwork.org.uk

CHAPTER 13

Inflammatory Bowel Disorders (IBDs)

Two inflammatory bowel disorders – ulcerative colitis (UC) and Crohn's disease – share similar symptoms and are generally grouped together under the umbrella term 'IBD'. Scientists don't yet know what causes either of them and it could well turn out that their causes are entirely different. They are not 'infectious' – people with either of these diseases cannot transmit them to others. IBDs affect an estimated 150,000 people in the UK, costing roughly £500 million a year in treatment and employee absence, according to the Association of the British Pharmaceutical Industry. Almost a third of this money is spent on the 2 per cent of IBD patients who suffer most severely.

Sometimes the acronym 'IBD' is confused with 'IBS' – which stands for Irritable Bowel Syndrome. IBS is entirely different from IBD, even though the symptoms of IBS can appear to be quite similar to some of those seen in IBD. The key difference is that with IBS there is generally no physical inflammation of the bowel walls and therefore no bleeding. (IBS is discussed in Chapter 12.)

Proctitis, an inflammation that occurs in the rectum, is essentially a form of UC that is limited to the lower part of the rectum. It is discussed along with the other inflammatory bowel conditions in Chapter 14.

Ulcerative Colitis (UC)

UC – sometimes loosely referred to as procto-colitis – is a disease that affects the inner lining of the colon and rectum (which together make up the large intestine), making it sore and inflamed. It sometimes causes ulcers to develop and bleed, and mucus and pus to be discharged into the bowel.

UC has similar symptoms to several other bowel problems, like Crohn's disease and IBS. However, diagnosis can usually be easily made by looking at a small tissue sample (biopsy) taken from the inflamed area of large intestine. UC sufferers tend to have quiet periods where the illness is dormant ('remissions'), interspersed with more active bouts of disease ('flare-ups').

About 25 per cent of UC sufferers also have problems with joint inflammation (like arthritis or ankylosing spondylitis) and occasionally eye inflammation (uveitis or iritis), as well as skin and liver problems. However, doctors still don't know how these problems are linked with UC and inflammatory bowel diseases in general.

UC slightly increases your chances of developing bowel (colorectal) cancer. The risk grows with both the severity and the duration of the disease and annual screening for bowel cancer is therefore normally advised once you have had UC for 8–10 years.

There are several theories about what may cause UC. See 'The IBD Detectives: Looking at Clues' on page 162.

Who can it affect? It affects males and females equally.

Incidence: UC affects around 100,000 people in Britain and an estimated 1 million people in the US. Worryingly, numbers seem to be increasing. UC is predominantly a disease of westernized countries, tending to affect those living in the northern hemisphere more than in tropical countries.

Age-bias: The disease most commonly starts between the ages of 15 and 35, but can occur at any age.

Risk factors:
- UC is more common among non-smokers and ex-smokers.
- Family links explain about 10 per cent of known cases.
- UC is also more common in certain ethnic groups, particularly people of Jewish descent.

Symptoms:
- Needing to visit the toilet *urgently* (often the worst symptom)
- Diarrhoea

- Bleeding
- Frequent need to visit the toilet
- Pus or mucus in the stools or from the rectum
- Occasional faecal incontinence
- When severe, the whole body can be affected, causing, in addition:
  - Abdominal pain
  - Tiredness and lethargy
  - Fever
  - Anaemia
  - Weight loss
  - Skin or eye irritations, arthritis and liver problems
  - Delayed growth and puberty (in children).

What can your doctor do?

- Early diagnosis can help, as several treatments seem to prolong periods of remission and reduce the frequency and severity of flare-ups.
- Medication:
  - 5-ASA drugs, a combination of sulphonamide sulphapyridine and/or salicylate (an aspirin derivative), can help control inflammation and seem to increase periods of remission. They include sulphasalazine (Salazopyrin), mesalazine (e.g. Asacol and Pentasa), olsalazine (Dipentum) and balsalazide (Colazide). They are often used first, as they are well tolerated long-term. Side effects may include nausea, vomiting, heartburn, diarrhoea, headaches and kidney damage.
  - Corticosteroids are often used to treat severe attacks of UC that have not responded to simpler medicines. These are anti-inflammatory drugs, which also tend to suppress the immune system. Prednisolone, prednisone and hydrocortisone can be taken as:
    - Tablets, suppositories, as an intravenous (IV) drip, or in foam or liquid retention enemas (i.e. medicine which is kept in the bowel for as long as possible – easier with a foam than a liquid!)
    - Long-term high-dose steroids. These are avoided where possible, because of the side effects, which include:
      - Weight gain
      - 'Moon face' – characteristic rounding of the face and cheeks
      - Increase in facial hair and acne, thinning of the skin

- High blood pressure (hypertension)
- Muscle weakness
- Mood changes/depression
- Thinning of bones (osteoporosis)
- Increase in blood sugar, occasionally triggering diabetes

Steroid drugs also lower immunity, making the patient more susceptible to infections like colds and flu. Steroid drugs should always be stopped gradually, never suddenly. For this reason, steroid cards should always be carried, in case the patient is involved in an accident or needs emergency treatment.

- A newer corticosteroid called budesonide has been introduced to treat mild UC. It appears to be almost as effective as corticosteroid drugs, but with fewer side effects.

- Immunosuppressant drugs: These work by damping down the immune system, which tends to have a similar effect in reducing the inflammation in bowel tissues. Drugs used for this purpose include azathioprine (Imuran), 6-mercaptopurine (Puri-Nethol) and ciclosporin (Sandimmun(e)). Ciclosporin may be used in the hospital treatment of acute and severe UC and requires close medical monitoring.

- Heparin: Used to prevent blood clots, heparin has shown promising results in the treatment of colitis, although most reports have been anecdotal rather than clinically proven. Heparin is routinely given to hospitalized patients taking IV prednisolone in order to prevent blood clots.

- Remicade (infliximab): This drug, which has been used to treat severe Crohn's disease, may in the future play a role in treating severe UC. It is an antibody that blocks an important inflammatory factor in the tissues. One study shows that the drug can induce positive responses in some patients. Further controlled studies are presently underway to see if the drug can usefully be added to the arsenal of medicines currently prescribed.

- Nicotine: There is some evidence that nicotine might be linked to UC. UC often affects non-smokers or ex-smokers and preliminary studies using nicotine therapy have shown promising results in improving symptoms.

- Folic acid and iron supplements may be prescribed as anaemia can result from the bleeding and general debilitation caused by UC.

- Surgery may be recommended if:
  - You suffer a severe attack that won't respond even to intensive hospital treatment. Occasionally, a sudden and severe attack may cause 'toxic megacolon'. This distends and may perforate the colon, which can lead to peritonitis, a medical emergency (see page 182).
  - The majority of your colon is affected, you are suffering from frequent and repeated attacks, and are generally not responding to medication. At this point your quality of life would be very poor and surgery is offered to improve it.
  - Your attacks are accompanied by inflammation in many other areas of your body – like the eyes, skin and joints, causing immobility and severe pain.
  - Doctors detect pre-cancerous or cancerous changes in your bowel walls.

  Surgical options are discussed in Chapter 18.

What can you do?
- Prevention: Because the cause of UC is not yet understood, there is little you can do to prevent the illness.
- Triggers: Try to avoid things that trigger flare-ups. These can include stress, diet (see dietary help, below), fatigue, certain drugs and antibiotics, even bouts of illness like colds and flu.
- Anti-diarrhoeal medication: Loperamide is often used to limit the diarrhoea that happens with UC, although it should not be taken without your doctor's advice. Bulking agents, like ispaghula husk (used in preparations like Fybogel and Isogel) can help thicken bowel output, which can sometimes relieve feelings of urgency and incomplete evacuation.
- Dietary help:
  - A low residue diet may be advisable.
  - Avoid any suspected dietary triggers – spicy curries affect some people; others find that milk, dairy or wheat products affect them.
  - Elemental or polymeric diets are occasionally used to good effect in UC (see section on Crohn's disease for details of elemental diets).
  - Soothing spices: IBD researchers are investigating turmeric, as it appears to help relieve inflammation. Ginger may have a similar effect.
- Visualization: Some studies suggest that visualization and imagery may play a role in improving UC. Imagine the ragged, ulcerated walls of the colon healing

and becoming smooth as you breathe deeply in a quiet environment and let yourself relax.

- Herbal help: Aloe vera juice is often reported as useful in soothing an inflamed bowel, and is widely available in health food stores. Slippery elm is also commonly used to help bowel inflammations.
- Reflexology: Many sufferers report that this helps alleviate symptoms. It's a good relaxing technique and may also help relieve associated joint pains.
- Relaxation techniques: Relaxation is useful if you suffer from stress, or suspect that stress is a trigger.
  - Indian head massage is a good total de-stressing treatment.
  - Aromatherapy massage is very good for general relaxation.
- Dealing with joint pains: Joint pain, often in the knees, wrists, shoulders, hips and back is an unfortunate and frequent accompaniment to UC. It is often mild, but can become severe and quite debilitating.
  - Many people take NSAIDs to alleviate joint pain. **However, always take care with NSAIDs (non-steroidal anti-inflammatory drugs like ibuprofen) as they can aggravate the symptoms of IBD.** Recent research by Professor Raymond Playford at Leicester General Hospital suggests that the health food supplement bovine colostrum may offer a cheap and effective way to prevent and treat the tissue damage associated with NSAIDs.
  - Yoga is useful for relaxation and meditation, but especially good for easing joint pain and improving mobility.
  - Aromatherapy massage can help improve muscle and joint stiffness.
  - Magnet therapy has also been reported as helpful in relieving joint pain and improving circulation.
- See Self-Help for Diarrhoea (page 14), Bleeding (page 20), Urgency, Frequency and Incomplete Evacuation (page 29), Mucus (page 21), and Abdominal Pain (page 24).

Further information:
The National Association for Colitis and Crohn's Disease (NACC), www.nacc.org.uk
Crohn's and Colitis Foundation of America (CCFA),
www.ccfa.org/medcentral/library/basic/facts1.htm
ibd Club, www.ibdclub.org.uk/
The Ileostomy and Internal Pouch Support Group, ia,
www.ileostomypouch.demon.co.uk

What is a Low-Residue Diet?

A low-residue diet is essentially the opposite of a high-fibre diet and is used where diarrhoea is a persistent problem. It eliminates excess fibre, which can irritate the bowel and aggravate inflammation, and leaves less waste for the bowel to deal with – and less waste should mean fewer bowel movements.

Don't Eat:

- Wholegrain cereals, pasta and bread
- Brown rice, pulses and beans
- Nuts and seeds
- Salads
- Skins and piths of fruit and potatoes
- Dried fruit
- Mushrooms, raw apples, sweetcorn and peas – all of which tend not to get chewed properly and are not very easily digested

Do Eat:

- Refined cereals and white bread
- Well cooked vegetables
- Cooked or canned fruit (without skins or seeds)
- 'Smooth-style' fruit and vegetable juices
- Tender meat, avoiding gristle
- Liquid food supplements (if necessary)

Tips:

- Chew food thoroughly before swallowing
- Eat small meals regularly instead of one or two large meals
- Try soups or purees
- Ask about bulking agents and stool softeners if constipation becomes a problem

Crohn's Disease

Crohn's disease (named after the American doctor Burrill Crohn, who described the illness in 1932) can potentially affect not just the large bowel (as in UC), but the small intestine and anywhere along the entire digestive tract from the mouth to the anus. Crohn's also differs from UC in that the inflammation typically affects the deeper layers of the intestinal walls, as well as the more superficial layers of the intestinal mucosa.

Crohn's disease is sometimes given the following names:

- Ileitis – when it affects the lower part of the small intestine
- Gastroduodenal Crohn's disease – when it affects the stomach and the first part of the small intestine
- Jejunoileitis – when it affects the jejunum and the ileum (the upper and lower portions of the small intestine)
- Ileocolitis – when it affects the ileum and colon (the most common form of Crohn's)
- Crohn's (granulomatous) colitis – when it affects the colon only

What effects does Crohn's disease have?
- Crohn's disease causes the intestinal walls to become inflamed. Sometimes they become thickened, which can cause a narrowing (stricture) of the affected part of the gut. In severe cases this can lead to obstruction or blockage of the intestine – a serious complication that normally requires surgery (see page 183).
- Sometimes the inflammation and damage penetrates so deep inside the gut walls that large openings or perforations form, called fistulae. These may cause gut contents to leak out through the skin around the anus, the bladder or the vagina. Fistulae sometimes discharge pus.
- Other complications of Crohn's include:
  - The development of anal fissures (see page 137)
  - Abscesses or boils around the anus (see page 134)
  - Skin 'tags' – painless lumps of skin that form around the anus
- People with Crohn's disease often suffer immune system abnormalities, for example arthritis, skin problems like erythema nodosum (painful red swellings,

153

usually on the legs, which fade leaving a bruise-like mark), inflammation of the eyes, and mouth ulcers.

- Crohn's sufferers are also prone to developing kidney stones, gallstones, or other diseases affecting the liver and gall bladder.
- Oral Crohn's, a rare form of the disease, causes swollen lips and, according to Professor David Wray at Glasgow Dental School, can be 'quite disfiguring'. Curiously, around 400 patients have been diagnosed with this rare condition in the west of Scotland over the last few years. (This compares to a mere 40 cases recorded in the whole of the US.) There are questions about whether there is a genetic predisposition to it in this area of Scotland and whether preservatives or flavourings in food may worsen the problem.

What causes Crohn's disease? Nobody knows what causes Crohn's disease. Some suspect that it is caused by a virus or bacteria, which triggers the immune system to respond by setting up inflammation deep inside the walls of the intestine.

Other research indicates that Crohn's may be caused by several factors – an over-reactive immune system, certain foods, environmental factors and perhaps other unknown variables. There may be a link with smoking: Crohn's disease is much more common in smokers than in non-smokers. See The IBD Detectives: Looking at Clues on page 162.

Who can it affect? Crohn's affects the sexes equally and there is a tendency for it to run in families. It is largely a disease of the developed world – mainly the US and Europe. It is also more common in urban populations than rural ones, and more common in northern compared to southern climates.

Incidence: Crohn's disease affects 30–40,000 people in the UK, with around 4,000 new cases being diagnosed each year. It affects an estimated 1,000,000 Americans. It does seem to be becoming more prevalent, especially among children.

Age-bias: Crohn's can happen at any age, but is most commonly diagnosed in people aged between the ages of 15 and 35.

Risk factors:

- Smoking – Crohn's affects smokers more than non-smokers.
- Inheritance – if you have a relative with Crohn's disease, your chances are up to 10 times higher than normal of developing Crohn's yourself, and up to 30 times if the relative is a sibling.
- Crohn's is more prevalent in certain ethnic groups, and very prevalent among Jewish people – Ashkenazi Jews are 4–5 times more likely to have IBDs than average.

Symptoms: These depend on which part of the gastrointestinal tract is involved and how it is being affected.

- Colitis-type symptoms:
  - Diarrhoea and occasional faecal incontinence
  - Weight loss
  - Bleeding
- Anal disease symptoms:
  - Anal pain (especially on opening the bowels)
  - Anal discharge
- Obstructional symptoms:
  - Colicky pain, often in the lower right corner of the abdomen
  - Abdominal distension
  - Weight loss
  - Vomiting
  - Diarrhoea
  - Occasionally constipation (if the disease has caused a narrowing in the small intestine)
- Fistulation or abscess symptoms:
  - Fever
  - Pain
  - Discharge
  - Weight loss
- Other general symptoms:
  - Tiredness and feeling 'unwell'
  - Anaemia
  - Delayed or stunted growth in children and delayed onset of puberty in pre-teens

What can your doctor do?

- Diagnosis is key, because then the disease can start to be controlled and its consequences – anaemia, malabsorption, weight loss and poor nutrition – can be remedied. This is especially important in children whose growth may suffer through inadequate nutrition.
- Symptomatic drugs can relieve some symptoms of Crohn's. They include:
  - Antidiarrhoeal medications: Loperamide (Imodium, Arret) or diphenoxylate (Lomotil) help relieve diarrhoea.
  - Rehydration salts: These restore the body's balance of fluids and vital salts that are lost through chronic or acute diarrhoea.
  - Cholestyramine: This 'resin' attaches itself to bile salts and can treat diarrhoea that is caused by the salts spilling into the large intestine from the ileum.
  - Bulking agents: These help relieve diarrhoea by providing more bulk, making the stool consistency thicker (and easier to pass).
  - Painkillers can relieve abdominal pain and joint pain that may accompany Crohn's disease. NSAIDs like ibuprofen (Brufen, Nurofen) are good anti-inflammatory painkillers, but they can make intestinal inflammation worse and must be used with caution. Paracetamol is often the safest drug to take.
  - Nutritional support may be needed if food is not being absorbed properly because of damage to the small intestine. Vitamin B12 injections are generally necessary if the lower end of the small intestine (the ileum) is affected. Folic acid and iron may also be prescribed. Other minerals and nutrients that may be depleted include calcium, salt, potassium, magnesium, vitamin D and zinc.
- Elemental and Polymeric diets: There is some evidence that simple food broken down to its basic nutritional components is more easily absorbed by a damaged digestive system, thus giving the intestines 'breathing space' to heal. Some experts claim significant success in getting their patients into remission using these diets. However, they're anything but 'gourmet' food and generally only the hardiest patients are able to tolerate them for more than a week or two at a time.
  - Elemental diets are given as a liquid taken through a straw or nasogastric feeding tube.

- Polymeric diets (e.g. Modulen) use larger molecules of nutrition, but omit all traces of indigestible fibre.
- Total Parenteral Nutrition (TPN): If the intestines are severely disturbed, then TPN can be given intravenously – it is a complete nutritive liquid that is taken directly into the bloodstream, allowing the intestines to 'rest' completely.
- Antibiotics:
  - Some experts believe that one cause of Crohn's disease is the bacterium *Mycobacterium Avium subspecies paratuberculosis*, or MAP. According to Professor John Hermon-Taylor at London's St George's Hospital Medical School, a combination of the antibiotics clarithromycin and rifabutin have shown a degree of success in treating Crohn's patients.
  - Crohn's sufferers are prone to developing abscesses due to overgrowth of certain bacteria. In such cases, antibiotics like metronidazole (Flagyl), vancomycin and ciprofloxacin are used.
- Anti-inflammatory drugs may be prescribed to reduce the inflammation in the gut, easing symptoms. These include:
  - 5-ASA drugs – In Crohn's disease, these drugs are often used to help lower the chances of the disease recurring following surgery to remove diseased portions of bowel. The drugs mesalazine (Asacol, Pentasa and Salofalk) tend to work as effectively in the small intestine as the colon.
  - Corticosteroids are normally given to treat acute attacks of the disease and are successful in about 80 per cent of cases. They help reduce inflammation in the intestines, as well as other affected areas like the joints, skin and eyes. There are side effects with long-term use and at higher doses. These include:
    - Increased appetite and weight gain
    - 'Moon' face and growth of facial hair
    - Acne
    - Raised blood sugar levels, which increases the risks of diabetes
    - High blood pressure
    - Mood swings
    - Weakening of the immune system, increasing the body's susceptibility to infections
    - Thinning of the skin and muscles and a tendency to bruise more easily
    - Osteoporosis

Anyone using high-dose steroids must carry a steroid card, and it is not advisable to stop treatment suddenly. Patients will be monitored carefully while on steroid medication.

- **Immuno-suppressant drugs:** These are most valuable when trying to 'wean' a patient off steroids, while still offering them protection against relapse. Originally developed to stop transplant patients from rejecting donor organs, they lower the immune response and, in doing so, tend to lower the inflammatory response that also causes IBD. They include the following:
  - **Azathioprine (Imuran) or 6-mercaptopurine (6-MP, or Puri-Nethol):** These drugs, often used in Crohn's patients, are slow-acting medicines that can take several months to achieve their effects. They may initially cause side effects including nausea or flu-like symptoms (aches and pains), and can affect the liver or the pancreas – though this is rare.
  - **Methotrexate:** This drug, mostly known as a cancer treatment, is also used to help relieve rheumatoid arthritis, another inflammatory disorder. It is often given with corticosteroids, because it appears to boost their effect, meaning that the patient doesn't have to take such high doses of steroids. Common side effects include nausea, vomiting, inflammation of the mouth and diarrhoea. It must not be taken by pregnant women or anyone trying to conceive.
  - **Remicade (Infliximab):** This monoclonal antibody blocks an important inflammatory substance and is the latest addition to the arsenal of medicines used to treat Crohn's. It is normally prescribed for severe cases where fistulas (abnormal channels that open up between the bowel walls and, say, the bladder, abdominal cavity or vagina) are occurring and where other treatments have failed. It seems to be effective in about two-thirds of patients but is expensive – each infusion costs about £2,000. Another drawback is that its effect is often short-lived. Almost all patients with fistulas who respond do later have recurrences of their fistula. Research is still ongoing as to how and when the drug is best used. The long-term safety profile remains to be established, although known side effects include nausea, headache and infections.
- **Thalidomide:** Despite its association with severe birth defects in the 1950s and 1960s, thalidomide has been investigated as an IBD treatment because of its potential to reduce the inflammatory response. It is approved for treating erythema nodosum (an uncommon complication associated with

Crohn's disease and leprosy) and there have been isolated reports of it helping people suffering from severe IBD where other drugs have failed.

- Interleukin-10 (IL-10): This is another immune system protein ('cytokine') that suppresses inflammation. Its efficacy in treating Crohn's is currently being investigated.
- Zinc: This mineral removes damaging free radicals (which may play a role in setting up inflammatory responses) from the bloodstream. Studies are ongoing to see if zinc supplements help reduce inflammation.

- Surgery is normally a last resort. Although surgeons can remove badly damaged sections of intestine, the disease can recur. If there is an intestinal blockage, a fistula, a severe abscess or bleeding, surgery may be necessary. If surgery involves the removal of a part of intestine well away from the anus, there is normally no need for a permanent stoma (where the intestine is brought out onto the surface of the abdomen into a bag, thus allowing waste to leave the body). A temporary stoma is made as a 'safety valve' above a surgical join (anastomosis) that can later be closed after the join has healed properly. If the anus has to be removed, there will be a permanent stoma. This will be either an ileostomy or a colostomy, depending on which part of the intestine it emerges from.

What can you do?
- Prevention: IBD is virtually unheard of in rural Africa and similar developing countries. Genetics aside, there are probably strong environmental influences. Diets high in unrefined cereals, grains and vegetables may offer some protection against IBD, whereas the Western diet, which is high in sugar, refined cereals, meat and dairy produce, may increase our chances of developing it.
- Stop smoking: Smoking increases the risk of developing Crohn's disease and it hampers the chances of successful recovery after surgery. It also increases the frequency and severity of disease flare-ups.
- Learn about Crohn's: There is a wealth of information available through self-help groups, information services, books and the Internet. Developments and breakthroughs are constantly being reported, and you can stay abreast of the latest knowledge by keeping informed. Knowledge is power and gives you a better sense of control. This way you are less likely to become overwhelmed or depressed about your condition.

- Dietary advice:
  - Some people find that certain triggers cause flare-ups. Dairy products and sugar are often cited, as are spicy foods, alcohol and wheat. Try to spot and avoid any potential food triggers.
  - Dr John Hunter at Addenbrooke's Hospital in Cambridge specializes in treating Crohn's disease using a programme of diet and nutrition. See Treating Crohn's with Food, opposite.
  - Try to eat good, wholesome foods that give your body the nutrition it needs and that will maintain your weight.
  - If you are suffering from a flare-up, avoid high-fibre foods and follow a low-residue diet to minimize digestive stress.
- Herbal help:
  - Mint tea or liquorice root tea, drunk daily, may help. Ginger juice is a natural anti-inflammatory.
  - Some complementary health experts advise taking 1 tsp psyllium husks in 5 tbsp natural live yoghurt mixed with 1 tsp Manuka honey, daily.
- Aromatherapy: Sesame oil massaged into the stomach may help ease pain and discomfort.
- Acupuncture: According to Mark Bovey, coordinator for the Acupuncture Research Resource Centre at Exeter University, several studies indicate that traditional acupuncture may offer a promising strategy for lowering disease activity and improving symptoms of Crohn's.
- Exercise: Assuming you are able, even gentle exercise can help the body produce natural steroids, as well as 'feel-good' endorphins. Try gently walking or swimming if you are suffering, but more vigorous activity and sport is better if you can manage it.
- See Self-Help for Nausea (page 17), Diarrhoea (page 14), Constipation (page 10), Bleeding (page 20), Abdominal Pain (page 24), and Urgency, Frequency and Incomplete Evacuation (page 29).

Further information:

National Association for Colitis and Crohn's Disease, www.nacc.org.uk

Crohn's & Colitis Foundation of America, www.ccfa.org

IBD Club – www.ibdclub.org.uk

The Ileostomy and Internal Pouch Support Group, ia, www.ileostomypouch.demon.co.uk

Treating Crohn's Disease with Food

Links between Crohn's disease and diet have long been suspected. Whatever those links may be, they seem to differ between individuals – which makes it very difficult to isolate the specific causes and therefore develop any universally effective treatments. Some experts suspect that sugar may be involved – several studies indicate that Crohn's disease sufferers eat more sugar than average. Fats, especially animal fats and polyunsaturated fatty acids (PUFAs), are also believed to play a role, according to much Japanese research (although omega-3 fats like EPA and DHA found in fish oils are believed to be beneficial to gut health). Even fibre is questioned, although the *source* of fibre (wheat versus vegetable fibre, for example) may be relevant. Even food colourings like titanium dioxide have been examined for a possible link to Crohn's disease.

Dr John Hunter, consultant gastroenterologist at Addenbrooke's Hospital in Cambridge, UK, specializes in treating Crohn's using a special programme of diet and nutrition. This involves an initial period (normally 2 weeks) of being fed an elemental diet (ED). Originally devised by scientists at NASA to give a convenient and complete source of nutrition, ED combines basic essential nutrients like amino acids, simple sugars, oils, minerals and vitamins. Because the diet is so simple, there is very little residue left by the time it enters the intestine. Dr Hunter says, 'We believe that Crohn's is caused by an immune reaction to the bacteria (flora) that live in the gut. Because the ED offers the flora nothing (in terms of residue or substrate) to feed on, it essentially "switches off" the fermentation activity of colonic flora. After 2 weeks on ED, the number of bacteria in the gut drops by 42 per cent.'

But ED is not gourmet food and the biggest reason for treatment failure is that some patients simply cannot tolerate the taste. 'Although palatability has been improved, about 15 per cent of patients cannot comply with the demands of ED,' he explains. 'However, there are significant benefits when you compare it to the alternative – corticosteroid treatment. ED is as effective in bringing patients into remission as steroid therapy. It also means that the serious side-effects of long-term steroid use are avoided – like that of developing osteoporosis.'

Dr Hunter follows the initial ED with a low-fat, fibre-limited exclusion diet (LOFFLEX), which avoids all the foods that are most likely to cause a relapse in the disease. 'The problem with ED is that symptoms generally recur as soon as the diet is stopped, but by following up with 2–4 weeks of LOFFLEX diet and then slowly reintroducing foods (omitting any that trigger symptoms along the way), over half of Crohn's patients can achieve long-term remission (up to 2 years or more) from active disease.'

The IBD Detectives: Looking at Clues

The causes of inflammatory bowel disease have eluded scientists for many years. They're not new illnesses – when Bonnie Prince Charlie fled to France in 1746, historians believe that his thinness and frailty was possibly due to UC. Inflammatory diseases don't just affect the bowels, either. The arthritis family of illness is characterized by inflammatory reactions and there are many links between arthritic conditions and IBDs – UC and ankylosing spondylitis (which affects the bones and typically the spine) often occur together. Research continues into genetics and the field of inflammatory physiology. Here are some of the key theories that attempt to explain why people develop UC and Crohn's disease.

MAP Bacteria

MYCOBACTERIUM AVIUM SUBSPECIES PARATUBERCULOSIS

Professor John Hermon-Taylor, a surgeon at London's St George's Hospital Medical School, has a special interest in microbiology and is a fervent believer that a cousin of the tuberculosis germ – called *Mycobacterium avium subspecies paratuberculosis* (MAP) – may be responsible for the majority of cases of Crohn's disease. Crohn's is prevalent in westernized society in temperate global regions and where there is intensive farming.

MAP bacteria are present in an estimated 7–55 per cent of dairy herds. They are hardy and hard-to-detect germs that infect cattle, sheep and goats, causing Johne's disease. Johne's disease is very similar to Crohn's disease in humans. Animals are very often infected sub-clinically, which means that although they are infected with MAP bacteria, they show no obvious symptoms or signs of disease. Hermon-Taylor believes that MAP can infect humans through contaminated milk and possibly even through the water supply, as a result of infected animals shedding faeces containing MAP onto farmland, where it enters the groundwater and rivers. The bacteria are tough enough to resist pasteurization at 72 degrees C for as long as 25 seconds, and have been found in a small number of pasteurized milk samples.

Hermon-Taylor says, 'We are facing a public health problem of tragic proportions – there are probably 90,000 people in Britain suffering from Crohn's disease and this figure will increase by around 5,000 every year. This insidious disease costs the health service nearly £300 million to treat annually, and ruins people's lives.' He believes it can sometimes be cured using antibiotics. 'We have refined techniques that have isolated MAP in the tissue of 94 per cent of patients tested who have Crohn's disease – this is highly significant. In addition, open clinical studies are showing that a half to three-quarters of Crohn's patients will improve if they are given a lengthy course of the antibiotics clarithromycin and rifabutin.'

More information is available through the Paratuberculosis Awareness & Research Association, www.crohns.org/para/index.htm

Conclusion: Although this theory is not yet accepted in mainstream medicine, it does put forward strong and persuasive arguments. Anyone especially worried about the possibility of MAP-contaminated milk should switch to either sterilized milk or soya milk.

Genetic Factors

'It's in the genes', they say. And perhaps it is. Scientists are always keen to explore the influences that genes have on health – whether the problem is cancer or even cellulite – and research into the possible genetic links with IBDs is no exception. For several years, various research units worldwide have linked Crohn's disease to human chromosome 16. Recent research by Professor Jack Satsangi at the Western General Hospital in Edinburgh (in collaboration with other international research teams) focused more precisely on the Nod2 gene on this chromosome. Derek Jewell, Professor of Gastroenterology at Oxford University's Nuffield Department of Medicine explains, 'Mutations of the Nod2 gene are clearly linked with the form of Crohn's disease that affects the small intestine. Mutations of this gene are present in up to 30 per cent of Crohn's cases and studies using identical twins also show there is an inheritable link to the disease. We are also beginning to see that other chromosomes may be involved – for example, Chromosomes 5 and 6 also seem to contain genes that may influence Crohn's disease.'

But is it *all* in the genes? Professor Jewell believes that although your genetic inheritance may be important in developing Crohn's disease, it probably doesn't fully explain it. 'The current model we are working on is that IBDs like UC and Crohn's disease are caused by an interaction between your genetic susceptibility and the environmental factors you meet. The evidence that there is a definite genetic influence is now incontrovertible,' he says. 'If you have an IBD there is roughly a 15 per cent chance that one of your family members will also have or develop it. What we now need to do is discover how these genes make people susceptible and look at their interaction with other environmental factors like smoking, diet, gut bacteria, previous use of antibiotics and even the use of NSAIDs'.

Conclusion: This is a rapidly expanding area of research – and several genes may be involved that influence the development of IBD. The strongest evidence so far points to links with Crohn's disease, although UC may also be influenced by genetic factors in similar ways.

Sulphate-Reducing Bacteria (SRBs)

The lower part of the gut – the colon – is teeming with bacteria. And as you travel from the right-hand side of the colon (where the small intestine empties into it) to the descending colon on the left-hand side, the activities of bacteria change dramatically. There is a theory that certain bacteria – specifically, the genus of bacteria called *Desulfovibrio* that produce toxic sulphur compounds – may be the cause or trigger of UC. According to Professor Glenn Gibson, these bacteria inhabit the colons of about 50 per cent of the human population, but 'sufferers of ... UC have a universal carriage of *desulfovibrios*'. These sulphate-reducing bacteria (SRBs) use sulphate, which is present in the diet, to metabolize organic materials to produce hydrogen sulphide, a gas that is both smelly and extremely toxic. SRBs can also 'feed' on the sulphur compounds found in proteins and preservatives, to make the toxin.

Research has shown that sulphated polymers fed to lab animals resulted in colitis-like lesions developing in the animals' guts, whereas this didn't happen if the animals had no bacteria in their colon at all. This strongly points towards the possibility that certain bacteria may be key agents in inflammatory disorders like UC, with SRBs the current favourites. It's also interesting to note that UC tends to start in the rectum and descending colon – where the greatest concentration of these bacteria are normally present – and only as the disease worsens does it travel further back along the colon toward the ascending colon and caecum. Furthermore, UC never affects the small intestine, which happens to have a different chemical environment and transit time, as well as far fewer resident bacteria. These factors would probably render the actions of sulphate-reducing bacteria ineffective.

Professor John H. Cummings, Professor of Experimental Gastroenterology at Ninewells Hospital Medical School in Dundee, has conducted much research in this area. He says studies show that people with untreated UC have higher levels of the toxic gas hydrogen sulphide in their colons than either treated patients or healthy people. He also notes that the drugs most commonly used to treat UC – 5-ASA drugs like mesalazine – are very good at stopping bacteria from producing this harmful gas. He is researching diets that limit the availability of sulphur compounds (like high-protein foods and preservatives). With such diets the SRBs have less to feed on and are less able to thrive and produce their toxic waste products.

Professor Gibson believes that altering the bacterial balance in the gut may help: if larger numbers of 'friendly' bacteria, like *bifidobacteria* and *lactobacilli* were introduced to the gut, they may help prevent a dominance of SRBs, thus reducing toxins and leading to less inflammatory damage.

Conclusion: The argument for bacterial involvement in UC seems strong, especially given that this disease is most often present (and limited) to the colon, which is where the suspect *Desulfovibrio* bacteria are found – and especially in the left side where UC starts. It is not advisable to avoid protein, but probiotic/prebiotic supplements that introduce or encourage the growth of larger numbers of 'friendly' bacteria may help.

Smoking

The link between smoking and IBD is an interesting one, because it appears to have opposite effects on Crohn's sufferers compared to UC patients.

Crohn's disease affects far more smokers than non-smokers and the symptoms also seem to be worse, with more frequent flare-ups in smokers than in non-smokers. Compared to non-smokers, smokers have double the risk of developing Crohn's. Young women are especially vulnerable, being between 4 and 10 times more likely to develop the disease as non-smokers. Given that there are more young women smoking in Britain than ever before, this is particularly worrying. Furthermore, in smokers, the effects seem to persist even after they've developed the disease. A Crohn's patient who has already had surgery has almost double the chances of having further surgery if they continue to smoke. However, it's not all cut and dried. Research in Israel, where there is a high incidence of Crohn's (which tends to affect Jewish people especially), finds no significant link with smoking.

Scientists can't yet explain why smoking seems to predispose people to having Crohn's disease. Nicotine may affect the way that blood circulates through the gut, or it may make the gut lining more susceptible to inflammation.

With UC, the observations are surprisingly different. Most UC patients don't smoke (only about 12 per cent of colitis sufferers smoke) and patients often report that their problems with UC developed soon after they had quit smoking. One gastroenterologist anonymously says, 'I often see patients with UC whose disease onset coincided with giving up smoking. Doctors generally won't openly acknowledge a link, because of the fear that people simply won't give up smoking in case they get UC but, let's face it, lung cancer, bronchitis, heart disease – these are all problems of epidemic proportions that are far more serious to health in the long run than colitis.' Absolutely.

And it's not that straightforward, anyway, so put away the ashtray and keep reading ... If you think that somehow smoking 'prevents' you from developing colitis, then you should note that while nicotine patches are sometimes useful in helping mild to moderate attacks of colitis, the use of nicotine as a *preventative* measure has so far shown no positive results. Furthermore, not everyone can tolerate nicotine: about 10 per cent of people given patches stop taking them because of side effects like nausea, headaches and giddiness. For more information about smoking and the digestive system, visit www.niddk.nih.gov/health/digest/pubs/smoke/smoking.htm

Conclusion: It appears that smoking is linked to Crohn's disease and UC, but in different ways. Stopping smoking appears to be a sensible choice for anyone, especially as it is implicated in the development of many cancers, heart disease and even problems like ulcers. But it is especially important if you have Crohn's disease. People with UC may find that nicotine treatment helps relieve mild bouts of the disease, but they should only try this therapy on their doctor's advice.

The MMR Vaccination

Over the last decade, the British press has been filled with stories about the possible links between the MMR vaccine routinely given to children in the UK and the development of autism and bowel problems resembling Crohn's disease. Dr Andrew Wakefield and colleagues at London's Royal Free Hospital, who investigated whether there was a link between the MMR vaccine and the onset of these developmental and digestive problems, conducted the original research. Since then, controversy has raged. According to the National Association for Colitis and Crohn's Disease (NACC), the original research did have methodological problems, which may cast doubt on the findings. Several other studies have failed to establish a link between the MMR and bowel or autism problems. But there are strong feelings among parent and other groups that there is 'more to this than meets the eye' and there are other studies that appear to support the original research. Meanwhile, the government and certain key medical establishments have urged parents not to let their children go unvaccinated because of what some have called 'scaremongering'.

The theory is that the measles virus may set up inflammation in the bowel walls, resulting in what appears to be Crohn's disease. If this were the case, then exposure to either the disease *or* the vaccine ought to provide triggers in susceptible people and there would therefore be no reason to avoid the vaccine, especially as measles can be fatal.

Some people worry that it is the 'three-in-one' nature of the MMR vaccination that proves too much for the child's developing immune system to handle all at once – hence the desire by many parents to have their children vaccinated singly, leaving reasonable spacing between each jab for the immune system to adapt and recover. Derek Jewell, Professor of Gastroenterology at Oxford University's Nuffield Department of Medicine, believes this is not a valid issue. 'There is no evidence suggesting that a single measles vaccine is any better or worse than the triple vaccine and the immune overload theory seems to derive from emotion rather than scientific fact. If single vaccines are given, then it will take over a year to get a child vaccinated properly – lots of needles and poor protection during that time.'

This is one of those unfortunate situations where conflicting medical views, politics and perhaps vested interests are all causing mayhem. Vaccination *is* an important social responsibility and unless a high percentage (95 per cent according to The World Health Organisation) of the population 'opt into' the vaccination policy, it will not ultimately work. However, parents have the right to protect their children from perceived risks and they certainly have a right to information. Many feel they are being denied this information and have not been offered persuasive reasons why single vaccinations are not widely available and are being discontinued by various key manufacturers. Even Dr Eileen Rubery, who chaired the committee that introduced the MMR vaccine in the UK, has now gone on record saying that offering parents the choice of single vaccines could end the stalemate that currently prevails. Unfortunately, all this confusion is to the detriment of only one thing – the prevention of serious illness. Professor Derek Jewell advises parents not to be unduly worried: 'As the evidence linking the MMR vaccine with Crohn's disease is even weaker than for autism, parents need to be reassured. Measles kills – we are all too young to have experience of this, but an epidemic in Afghanistan killed thousands only two years ago. Children can develop problems without having measles or the MMR and many surveys have shown that the introduction of the vaccine has not coincided with a major increase in autism.'

Conclusion: This contentious issue doesn't appear close to being resolved. Scientific evidence that supports the MMR vaccine has been undermined by other studies and reports, and by a high-profile campaign against it. If any kind of vaccination programme is to survive, it must have the confidence and cooperation of parents, which the MMR programme has failed (of late) to achieve. Any family that already has exposure to bowel illness may be justifiably concerned about the possible effects of vaccinating their child (given the already higher risk of bowel illness developing in their offspring) and would have a valid argument for wanting to seek either single jabs, or avoiding the measles vaccine altogether.

CHAPTER 14

Other Inflammatory Gut Conditions

While UC and Crohn's disease are known as the two classic inflammatory bowel diseases, several other gut problems are also caused by inflammation – these are discussed here.

Gastritis

Gastritis simply means 'inflammation of the stomach lining'. It can be caused by:

- A viral or bacterial infection like food poisoning
- Infection with *Helicobacter pylori* bacteria
- Excess alcohol
- Smoking
- Aspirin use (or overuse)
- Certain anti-inflammatory painkillers (like ibuprofen)
- Some other prescription drugs

Who can it affect? Anyone, although children are normally only affected by viral or bacterial gastritis.

Incidence: Gastritis accounts for over 2 million visits to doctors' surgeries every year in the US.

Age-bias: None known.

Risk factors:

- Smoking
- Excess alcohol
- Too much caffeine
- Overeating
- Stress
- Use of non-steroidal anti-inflammatory drugs (NSAIDs) or aspirin

Symptoms:

- Abdominal pain or discomfort
- Nausea and vomiting (which occasionally may have the appearance of 'coffee grounds', indicating bleeding)
- Appetite loss
- Abdominal bloating
- Belching
- Hiccoughs
- Occasionally fever or fatigue

What can your doctor do?

- Viral gastritis is normally self-limiting and resolves itself within 24–48 hours. There is no treatment for it, other than keeping well hydrated, resting and avoiding food for 24 hours until symptoms start to settle.
- Bacterial gastritis responds well to antibiotics, and your doctor will be able to identify the likely cause.
- If you are taking aspirin or NSAIDs, stop taking them immediately, unless they have been prescribed for you, in which case contact your doctor or pharmacist for advice.
- Your doctor can do a test to see if your problem is caused by *H. pylori* infection.

What can you do?

- Avoid alcohol.
- Stop smoking.
- If you feel that stress aggravates your symptoms, adopt a regime of stress-relieving exercises like yoga or Pilates, or simply take up some form of exercise.

- Dietary help:
  - Avoid caffeineated and fizzy drinks, and milk, which can increase acid secretions in the stomach. Otherwise, drink plenty of water and fluids.
  - Eat more bland foods and avoid citrus fruit and fried, fatty foods.
- Herbal help: Chamomile tea and liquorice extract can both help.
- Vitamin boosters: Zinc and vitamin A supplements can help heal the stomach lining.
- See Self-Help for Nausea (page 17) and Abdominal Pain (page 24).

Further information:
Lebanon Health, www.lebanonhealth.com/condi/320.htm

Peptic Ulcers (Gastric and Duodenal Ulcers)

Peptic ulcers develop when the sensitive lining of the stomach and duodenum becomes ulcerated or inflamed – generally as a result of excess acid production in the stomach or the presence of the *Helicobacter pylori* bacterium. Peptic ulcers can occur either in the stomach (gastric ulcers) or in the duodenum, the upper part of the small intestine (duodenal ulcers).

Who can they affect?
- Peptic ulcers are almost always associated with infection by the bacterium **Helicobacter pylori. H. pylori** is present in virtually all those suffering from duodenal ulcers and about 80 per cent of people with gastric ulcers.
- Peptic ulcers affect one in 10 men and one in 15 women at some time and although they are not caused by stress, stress can make them worse.

Age-bias: They are more common in the over-30s.

Risk factors: The following may cause ulcers or aggravate existing ones:
- Smoking
- Alcohol (especially spirits)
- Aspirin and certain anti-inflammatory (NSAID) drugs

Symptoms:

- Pain, normally felt near the stomach, occasionally spreading between the ribs and through to the back.
- The pain is often 'burning', can be relieved by eating and may be worse at night.
- Occasionally, a peptic ulcer can cause vomiting.

What can your doctor do?

- *H. pylori* infection is known to cause ulcers in the vast majority of those infected with it. It can be tested for in several ways including blood, breath or stool tests, or with tissue samples obtained by endoscopy.
- *H. pylori* infection is usually treated with antibiotics.
- Antacid medicines may also be suggested to neutralize the stomach acids.
- Other drugs that may be prescribed include ulcer-healing drugs, which reduce the secretions produced by the stomach. They include proton pump inhibitor (PPI) medicines like omeprazole (Losec), and H2 receptor antagonist drugs like cimetidine (Tagamet and Peptimax) and ranitidine (Zantac). Other drugs like misoprostol (Cytotec) and bismuth may occasionally be used.
- Endoscopy (where a flexible tube containing a camera is swallowed by the patient) allows the doctor to closely examine the stomach lining and identify any ulcers or patches of inflammation and soreness. It also helps to rule out more serious conditions like stomach cancer.
- With treatment, 95 per cent of ulcers disappear completely within a month, although they do tend to recur if 'bad' habits (like smoking or drinking) persist, or if reinfection with *H. pylori* occurs.

What can you do?

- Don't smoke. Smoking aggravates ulcers. It is believed that cigarettes cause the body to overproduce stomach acid. Because smoking acts as an appetite suppressant for many people, smokers are also more likely to skip meals.
- Avoid alcohol. Alcohol (especially spirits) irritates the stomach lining and although it rarely causes ulcers, it can make existing ulcers worse (or increase the likelihood of them developing).
- Cut down on caffeine. It is also a suspected aggravating factor.
- Avoid aspirin and anti-inflammatory drugs, as these can also inflame the stomach lining. If you need aspirin or NSAIDs, your doctor can give you a

proton pump inhibitor drug to take with them. Paracetamol is a safe alternative painkiller.

- Don't rush your meals and avoid diets that are high in fat, salt and sugar, but low in fibre.
- Introducing 'friendly flora' into the gut may help. Take probiotics regularly, either as live yoghurt, yoghurt-based drinks or tablets.
- Pepto-Bismol contains bismuth subsalicylate, which is known to kill *H. pylori* and protect the stomach lining.
- Herbal help: Meadowsweet is an antacid that soothes the stomach. Slippery elm soothes and protects the digestive tract. Both herbs are known and used for their anti-ulcer effects.
- See Self-Help for Nausea (page 17), and Abdominal Pain (page 24).

Further information:
Diagnosis Health.com, www.diagnosishealth.com/ulcer.htm
The Helicobacter Foundation, www.helico.com

Proctitis

Proctitis is inflammation in some or all of the rectum. It is sometimes confused with haemorrhoids because the symptoms of bleeding, pain and mucus discharge can be identical, although there is nothing protruding from the anus. Because internal haemorrhoids – where nothing protrudes from the anus – are more common than external haemorrhoids, it can be hard to tell the difference without examining the area with a proctoscope. (You can also have both haemorrhoids and inflammation, confusing the picture further.)

What causes it?
- Proctitis occurs in ulcerative colitis (UC) and in many cases of Crohn's disease, but can also be caused by any infection in the lining of the rectum. See Chapter 13 for more information on UC and Crohn's disease.
- Anal intercourse increases the risk of catching sexually transmitted infections like gonorrhoea, syphilis, chlamydia, cytomegalovirus or herpes simplex. These can cause proctitis.
- Proctitis can be caused by amoebic dysentery (amoebiasis) – see page 112.

- It can also be caused by radiotherapy treatment for cancer in the area near the rectum and anus. Men having radiotherapy for prostate cancer commonly get proctitis.

Who can it affect?
- People with UC and Crohn's disease
- Anyone engaging in anal intercourse
- Cancer patients undergoing radiotherapy in the lower abdominal area

Incidence: According to the *Merck Manual of Medical Information*, proctitis is becoming increasingly common.

Age-bias: None known, except it rarely occurs in children.

Risk factors:
- Genetics – Proctitis, a localized form of IBD, tends to run in families.
- Ethnicity – In the US, statistics show that Jews of European descent are 4–5 times more likely to develop IBDs (especially Crohn's disease) than average.
- Location – Proctitis is more prevalent in developed countries, more common in urban populations than rural ones, and more prevalent in northern climates.
- Anal intercourse, as this increases the chances of an infection (one that may result in proctitis), and may also lead to physical injury of the rectum.
- Radiotherapy used to treat cancers that are located near the rectum can also cause a form of proctitis.

Symptoms:
- Mucus or pus in the stools or from the rectum
- Bleeding in the stools or from the rectum
- Discomfort and pain in the back passage
- Feeling strong urges to defecate, occasional faecal incontinence
- Breaking 'wet wind'
- Cramps on the left side of the abdomen
- Constipation or diarrhoea
- Itching

If you have some or all of the symptoms listed above, visit your doctor. Proper treatment is important.

What can your doctor do?

- If the cause is UC or Crohn's, relevant drugs may be given (see Chapter 13) like Proctofoam, Colifoam or Predfoam (steroid-based foam enemas that may reduce local inflammation) or sulfasalazine drugs.
- Corticosteroids may ease the problem if it's caused by radiotherapy.
- Antibiotics are normally used if the cause is an infection.

What can you do?

- Although diarrhoea is the most common problem, constipation may occasionally occur. If it does, stool softeners or laxatives may help, but check with your doctor first.
- Avoid anal intercourse and sexual play, especially if the cause is an STI or physical injury.
- Tell your partner(s) if the cause is an infection, because it is important that they are treated too.
- Keep the area clean and dry – wash after every bowel movement and *gently* pat dry.
- Proctitis tends to have periods when it is active (often called 'flare-ups' or 'exacerbations') interspersed with quiet or inactive periods ('remissions'); triggers associated with flare-ups include stress, food and illness or being run-down. Try to isolate your triggers and avoid them. Sometimes it isn't very easy, especially if stress affects you.
- Painkillers can relieve any discomfort.
- Herbal help: Slippery elm tea is used to help relieve bowel distress.
- Avoid food and drink that may cause irritation, for instance beer, tea, coffee, milk, colas, tomatoes, citrus fruit, chocolate, spicy and peppery foods. Experience will tell you what to avoid.
- See Self-Help for Mucus (page 21), Bleeding (page 20), Pain in the Back Passage (page 25), Urgency, Frequency and Incomplete Evacuation (page 29), Abdominal Pain (page 24), and Itchy Bottom (page 31).

Further Information:

The ibd Club, www.ibdclub.org.uk

National Association for Colitis and Crohn's Disease, NACC, www.nacc.org.uk

Merck Manual of Medical Information – Home (Internet) Edition, www.merck.com/pubs/mmanual/section3/chapter35/35g.htm

Diverticular Disease

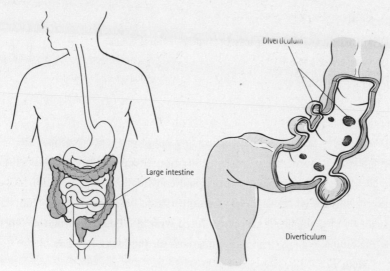

Large intestine

Diverticulum

Diverticulum

The intestinal walls are made of muscle. When a person is constipated, com-pacted bowel contents push against the muscular walls and, eventually, weak spots can occur – it's a little bit like the inner tube of a bicycle tyre that bulges out if it's overblown or weakened. The pouches that bulge out of the colon are called *diverticula* and when a person develops these (many do, particularly in industrialized countries) they are said to have *diverticulosis* or *diverticular disease*.

Diverticulitis happens when one or more of the diverticula become infected – this can be because of trapped waste matter, or because of bac-terial overgrowth leading to infection (somewhat similar to appendicitis). About 10–25 per cent of people with diverticulosis develop diverticulitis at some stage and it can recur.

Who can it affect?

- Diverticular disease is extremely common in developed societies, probably as a result of low-fibre diets that cause chronic, long-term constipation. It is very rare in continents like Africa, where people eat high-fibre diets and virtually no refined foods.
- Very rarely, people are born with a diverticulum in the small intestine.

Age-bias: Because diverticula develop slowly, older age groups are more likely to have them. Over half of all Brits and Americans aged over 70 have them.

Risk factors:
- Low-fibre diet containing lots of highly-refined foods
- Chronic constipation
- Chronic dehydration

Symptoms:
- Diverticulosis doesn't normally cause any symptoms – many people are completely unaware they have the condition. Some patients occasionally report feeling mild cramps, bloating and constipation.
- Diverticulitis – which happens when diverticula become infected – can start suddenly or gradually. It can be confused with IBS. Common symptoms include:
  - Abdominal cramps, pain and tenderness on the lower left side of the abdomen
  - Fever and chills
  - Nausea and occasionally vomiting
  - Alternating constipation and diarrhoea, sometimes just constipation
  - Occasionally, bright red bleeding from the back passage

What can your doctor do?
- Diverticulosis is often picked up during investigations for other problems.
- A simple digital rectal exam can often detect tenderness, blockages or bleeding that may accompany diverticulitis.
- Barium contrast x-rays, which involve an enema of radioactive barium followed by x-rays, can show up diverticular pouches in the intestine walls.
- Colonoscopies, ultrasounds and CT scans may also locate diverticula.
- If diverticular disease is detected early, often a simple dietary change (which involves increasing your fibre intake) may be all that is needed.
- If you get stomach cramps or abdominal pain, your doctor can prescribe pain relief or anti-spasmodic drugs to help, like Colofac or propantheline (Pro-Banthine).
- Motility stimulants (medicines that help the contents of the intestine move) like metoclopramide (Maxolon, Primperan) and cisapride (Alimix and Prepulsid) may occasionally help.

- For acute diverticulitis, a hospital stay may be necessary, where intravenous fluids and antibiotics will be given. In the majority of cases surgery isn't necessary.
- If there is bleeding or recurrent attacks of diverticulitis, there is a greater chance that surgery may eventually be needed. Normally, surgery involves removing the affected section of large bowel and reconnecting the remaining portions. Sometimes a temporary colostomy is needed while the reconstructed area heals (see Chapter 18, Hospitals, Surgery and More ...).
- Occasionally, a diverticulum can burst causing peritonitis (see page 182) or an abscess (page 134).
- Fistulas are a rare complication of diverticulitis – and can occur between the intestinal wall and the bladder or vagina, causing urinary problems or faecal discharge through the vagina.
- Another rare complication of diverticulitis is an intestinal blockage (see page 183).

What can you do?
- Prevention: This is key to avoiding diverticular disease – and is simple. Eat plenty of fibre, drink plenty of fluids and don't become chronically constipated.
- Dietary help:
  - Increase the amount of fibre In your diet.
  - Take fibre-drinks like Fybogel, Regulan, Metamucil or Citrucel.
  - Some doctors advise against eating any foods with small seeds that might lodge in the diverticula and lead to infection – like tomatoes, figs and strawberries. However, there is no firm evidence indicating that seeded foods do cause problems.
- See Self-Help for Constipation (page 10), Abdominal Pain (page 24), Nausea (page 17), Diarrhoea (page 14), and Bleeding (page 20).

Further information:
National Digestive Diseases Information Clearinghouse,
www.niddk.nih.gov/health/digest/pubs/divert/divert.htm
Digestive Disorders Foundation,
www.digestivedisorders.org.uk/Leaflets/divertnew.html

CHAPTER 15

Emergency Conditions

While the vast majority of health problems that people face are minor, there are occasions when seeking immediate medical help is vital. This section deals with the most common gut problems needing emergency treatment.

Appendicitis

Appendicitis is essentially an inflammation of the blind-ended, finger-sized tube that spurs off the large intestine (colon). The appendix is an anatomical relic from when our ancestors ate more vegetable matter and fibre than we do today, and seems to perform no discernible function whatsoever in modern man.

Having appendicitis doesn't necessarily mean you'll be whisked into hospital and put under the knife. You can get what doctors call a 'grumbling appendix', which causes recurrent phases of mild to moderate discomfort, but doesn't reach the acute stage of infection that necessitates its removal.

Suspected appendicitis should be attended to immediately, as peritonitis (which happens if the appendix bursts) can be fatal.

Who can it affect? It affects males slightly more than females, although it can be harder to diagnose in adult women – mainly because the ovaries, uterus and fallopian tubes also occupy the same area as the appendix.

Incidence: Appendicitis is a very common acute illness; we have a 7 per cent chance of being affected by it during our lifetime.

Age-bias: It's more common in children, teenagers and the elderly than it is in adults in their middle years.

Risk factors: Ovarian cysts, ectopic pregnancies and uterine or ovarian infections can cause symptoms similar to appendicitis and although CT scans, ultrasound scans and laparoscopies are regularly used to confirm a diagnosis, research from the University of Washington in Seattle shows that the rate of *misdiagnosis* is as high as 23.2 per cent among women patients, compared with only 9 per cent for male patients. So while being female doesn't make you more likely to develop appendicitis, women may be more likely to be wrongly diagnosed with it.

Symptoms: These vary between individuals, but generally develop over a few hours. Typical symptoms include:
- Intermittent pain in upper abdomen or around navel, gradually shifting to the lower right quadrant of the abdomen
- Nausea and sometimes vomiting
- Mild fever
- Loss of appetite
- Frequent urination and possibly diarrhoea

What can your doctor do?
- Appendicitis can't be prevented, but early diagnosis lowers the chance of complications like peritonitis.
- Because the appendix doesn't perform any obvious function, most doctors err on the side of caution and remove it if there is more than a reasonable chance that it is causing the problem.

What can you do? Not a lot – but see your doctor quickly if you suspect appendicitis. Children are more prone to appendicitis, so suspect it if your child complains of a bad 'tummy ache' – especially if it is accompanied by fever, vomiting or diarrhoea.

Further information:
National Digestive Diseases Information Clearinghouse,
www.niddk.nih.gov/health/digest/summary/append/index.htm

Kids Health for Parents,
http://kidshealth.org/parent/infections/stomach/appendicitis.html

Peritonitis

Peritonitis occurs when the peritoneum, the thin membrane that contains the abdominal organs, becomes inflamed. This can happen as a result of bacterial infection, or because of partly-digested food, digestive juices, blood or faeces that have leaked from abdominal organs – for example, a burst appendix, a ruptured ulcer or diverticulum, or an injury that pierces the abdominal area.

Who can it affect? Peritonitis can affect anyone, although men are slightly more susceptible.

Incidence: Peritonitis is rare and generally occurs as a complication of another illness – for example, fistulating Crohn's disease, appendicitis and perforated ulcers. It can also happen to people using certain forms of kidney dialysis and those with cirrhosis of the liver.

Age-bias: None known.

Risk factors:
- Any untreated condition that affects the abdomen – like appendicitis, burst ulcer, injury, pelvic inflammatory disease (PID), or a rupture of an ectopic pregnancy (one that implants into the fallopian tube and eventually ruptures the tube as it grows).
- There is a risk of peritonitis after abdominal surgery, due to infection. Peritonitis may also occur if a surgical join between two sections of intestine leaks.

Symptoms:
- Abdominal pain – normally starting quite suddenly, and increasing in severity. It is normally most intense near the site where the underlying cause is, for example, a burst appendix.
- Nausea and vomiting

- Fever and chills
- Rapid, thready heartbeat
- Low blood pressure
- Dizziness and weakness, and rapid breathing
- Shoulder pain (occasionally)
- Abdominal swelling

Peritonitis is a serious medical emergency. Call your doctor immediately if you suspect it.

What can your doctor do?
- Urgent treatment of the condition that has caused the peritonitis is essential. Treatment includes antibiotics to combat the infection and pain relief as necessary.
- Intravenous fluids and nutrition are given so that the intestinal tract can heal.

Further information:
MDAdvice, www.mdadvice.com/library/ped/pedillsymp315.html

Intestinal Obstruction or Intestinal Blockage

Intestinal obstructions and blockages occur when the passage of waste matter through the bowel is impeded or stopped for some reason. Intestinal obstructions can be complete or partial. Several things can cause an intestinal blockage:

- A strangulated hernia
- Adhesions
- Occasionally, intestinal muscles fail to contract properly and push waste through the intestines, as a complication of either peritonitis or major surgery.
- Tumours
- Both Crohn's disease and diverticular disease can also cause intestinal obstruction.

Who can it affect? Anyone, although intestinal obstruction is uncommon.

Age-bias: None.

Risk factors: These depend on the specific cause of the obstruction.

Symptoms: These can start suddenly or come on gradually, depending on the cause of the obstruction. They include:

- Severe constipation
- Vomiting – greenish–yellow or brown and smelling of faeces
- Abdominal bloating
- Pain, either 'colicky' (i.e. in waves) or continuous
- A total absence of wind or faeces being passed

Call your doctor urgently, as intestinal obstruction needs emergency treatment and will not respond to self-help or home remedies.

What can your doctor do?
- Intravenous fluids and nasogastric suction may be necessary.
- If the obstruction is caused by inflammation, drugs to treat this may help relieve the problem.
- Surgery is needed in some cases, and has a high success rate. See Chapter 18, Hospitals, Surgery and More ...

CHAPTER 16

Cancers and Growths

Under normal, healthy circumstances, body cells live for a while, perform their specific function, replicate themselves and eventually die – the medical word for cell death is 'apoptosis'. Cell death is pre-programmed and is a normal part of the cell's lifecycle. However, sometimes cells fail to die – instead, they keep replicating in an uncontrolled fashion until eventually an overgrowth, or tumour, occurs.

Growths come in two sorts – benign and malignant. Cancers are malignant and tend to spread locally, or they can migrate from their original site and set up shop elsewhere in the body. Doctors refer to these as 'secondaries', or 'metastases'. This is what has happened when a cancer has spread to a person's liver or bones, for example.

Because benign growths and malignant cancers are both caused by the abnormal proliferation of cells, they are discussed together in this section.

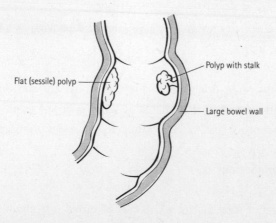

Flat (sessile) polyp

Polyp with stalk

Large bowel wall

Polyps

Polyps are abnormal projections of tissue that develop on the flat surface of the large bowel. They can be different shapes – either raised areas a little like moles, like mushrooms on stalks, or even like a 'carpet' of small finger-like projections. They tend to grow slowly, can occur either singly or in groups and vary in size from being a few millimetres to several centimetres. Scientists have not yet pinpointed the cause of polyps.

Some polyps are identified as 'adenomas' after microscope analysis. Adenomas may occur in certain rare inherited disorders such as Familial Adenomatous Polyposis (FAP) and Hereditary Non-Polyposis Colorectal Cancer (HNPCC). With FAP and HNPCC, adenomas are highly likely to become cancerous; people with these conditions should be monitored and their children screened for the disease.

Who can they affect? Polyps can affect either sex.

Age–bias: Polyps become more common with increasing age – as many as 1 in 3 people over the age of 60 may have them.

Incidence: Polyps are common, especially among people in developed countries.

Risk factors:
- A family history of bowel cancer, FAP or HNPCC.
- Stony Brook University researchers have identified smoking as a key risk factor for colorectal polyps.

Symptoms: Polyps often don't cause any symptoms and are only picked up during a routine test or health check, or when a bowel examination is performed for some other reason. When they do cause symptoms, these include:

- Bleeding from the anus
- Diarrhoea
- Some polyps ooze clear mucus, which may be mixed with stools.

- Very rarely, a large (normally malignant) polyp may cause an intestinal obstruction (see page 183), which leads to constipation, abdominal pain, bloating and vomiting.

What can your doctor do?
- In the majority of cases, polyps are discovered on x-ray (barium enemas) or colonoscopy.
- Most polyps are easily and painlessly removed by using a colonoscope – a flexible tube with a camera and small looped wire that is inserted into the colon. The wire, which becomes very hot, is placed round the polyp and burns it off. This procedure, called diathermy, is painless because there are virtually no nerve endings in the gut. Occasionally large polyps have to be removed surgically.
- All polyps are routinely examined for signs of cancer, though the *vast majority* are benign adenomas. If a cancerous polyp (adenocarcinoma) is found, you will be monitored to make sure that any recurrence is picked up early.
- If you have had an adenoma, you will probably be checked at regular intervals.
- People with FAP grow large numbers of adenomas and are also at very high risk of developing bowel cancer, although if no polyps have developed by the age of 40, it is generally unlikely that they will develop at all.
- The drug sulindac (normally used for arthritis) is sometimes used to reduce polyp development, although recent research from Johns Hopkins Kimmel Cancer Center casts doubt on the drug's ability to prevent polyps developing in patients with FAP.

What can you do?
- Since it is very common for polyps to go completely unnoticed, there is little anyone can do to prevent them.
- If FAP runs in your family, you must tell your doctor as you will need screening and monitoring.
- See Self-Help for Bleeding (page 20), Diarrhoea (page 14), and Mucus (page 21).

Further information:
The Polyposis Registry www.polyposisregistry.org.uk/FAPintro/whatisFAP.asp
Digestive Disorders Foundation,
www.digestivedisorders.org.uk/Leaflets/polypsnew.html

Colorectal (Large Bowel) Cancer

'As you get older, you have less energy – so when I started feeling tired I put it down to the fact that I was approaching my fifties. I've always had a tendency – like many women – to be constipated, but then I suddenly started getting loose bowel movements, sometimes several times a day, and often nothing much would even come out. One afternoon I heard a radio programme about bowel cancer, urging people not to be shy about their problems, and because my father died of bowel cancer in his sixties, I thought I ought to put my embarrassment behind me and see my GP. He arranged a FOB test and, after examining me, he said he could feel something, and referred me to a specialist. By this time I was feeling groin pain and losing weight.

The diagnosis was – even though I was steeling myself for it – still a shock, but the good news was that my cancer was picked up very early and was completely removed with surgery. I didn't need chemotherapy, and was feeling so much better even within a couple of weeks.

I did worry that I'd not be able to "finish" my job as a mother and see my children grow up. Now, three years after my diagnosis, I'm beginning to relax about my body again, and feel confident that I've beaten bowel cancer. I am so pleased that I listened to people's advice and saw my doctor early enough.'

Diana, 53, whose early stage bowel cancer was diagnosed three years ago

Colorectal cancer is so-called because the cells lining the colon and rectum are similar and therefore cancers that develop in this part of the digestive system are grouped together. (Cells lining the anal canal and anus are different and susceptible to different types of cancer, which is why anal cancer is discussed separately – see page 197).

Colorectal cancers normally start as adenomas that develop on the inner wall of the colon or rectum and grow out of control. Adenomas become increasingly common with age – about 25 per cent of people have at least one by the time they reach their fifties, but less than 10 per cent of them eventually become cancerous (malignant).

People with the rare inherited conditions FAP and HNPCC are at high risk of developing bowel cancer, although together they account for less than 5 per cent of all large bowel cancers. Low-fibre diets, diets high in animal fat and protein, a lack of exercise, sedentary occupations and smoking may also play a role.

Scientists know that certain genes may place some people at greater risk of developing colorectal cancers. Pioneering work by Professor David Lane, one of the scientists who discovered the p53 gene, has shown that this gene functions as a 'brake' on cells, stopping them from dividing uncontrollably. Up to 60 per cent of all cancers seem to be associated with a defective or damaged p53 gene, and additional genes are now being identified. Cancer Research UK has found, for example, that women with a damaged BRCA1 gene (which gives women a high risk of developing breast cancer) also have an increased risk of other cancers, including colon cancer. New research from Glasgow's Beatson Institute has identified a protein molecule called Src that plays a key role in loosening the tissue structures around a tumour, allowing cancer cells to spread more easily around the body.

Who can it affect?
- Anyone – colorectal cancer is one of the most common cancers. More than half a million cases are diagnosed worldwide each year, of which more than 30,000 are in the UK. Bowel cancer (as colorectal cancer is very commonly called) is also one of the biggest cancer killers – responsible for over 70,000 deaths in the US every year – and is the second leading cause of cancer death in Britain, accounting for 11 per cent of cancer deaths annually. The good news is that the cure–rate (for all bowel cancers and from all causes) is high if diagnosis is made early.
- Rectal cancer tends to be more common in men, while colon cancer is more common in women.
- Anyone with a history of polyps in the colon, especially if they are caused by the inherited condition FAP.

Age-bias: Colorectal cancer is not commonly found in the under-40s (less than 3 per cent of cases occur in this age group) but becomes increasingly common in the over-60s.

Risk factors:

- Genetics – Some people are more at risk because of their genetic inheritance, although only about 1 in 50 cases of bowel cancer have a genetic link.
- High-fat, low-fibre diets – Many studies suggest that because such foods typically take longer to pass through the gut than high-fibre diets, digestive waste is in contact with the bowel walls for far longer, allowing more contact between bowel cells and cancer-causing chemicals in the waste. Colorectal cancer is relatively rare where there are predominantly vegetarian diets or where less dietary fat is eaten – for example, in Japan. The incidence of colorectal cancer is far higher in countries where animal fats and proteins are consumed in large amounts – for example in New Zealand, Argentina and the US.
- Inflammatory bowel disease – If you have colitis or Crohn's disease, there is an increased risk that you may *eventually* develop bowel cancer. This is especially true if the disease has been active for more than 10 years. Most people with IBD do not, however, develop bowel cancer.
- Lack of exercise
- Excessive alcohol consumption
- Obesity – Canadian research shows that women who are clinically obese are twice as likely to develop bowel cancer before their menopause. This may be because excess body fat is associated with higher levels of blood insulin and related chemicals, which research has also linked to higher risks of bowel cancer.
- Radiation exposure to the pelvis or abdomen increases the risks, but not normally until 10–50 years after the exposure.

Symptoms: Often in the early stages there may be few or no symptoms. When they do appear, they may include:

- Blood on the surface of bowel motions – either red, dark red, or even blackish streaks of old blood – or passing mucus
- Diarrhoea or constipation that won't respond to self-help
- Changes in bowel habit such as unusual periods of diarrhoea or constipation that persist for more than a couple of weeks
- Feelings of incomplete emptying of the bowel (this is also very common with IBS)

- Unexplained anaemia (causing tiredness) and loss of appetite
- Colicky abdominal pain and/or tenderness
- If a tumour is causing a partial blockage of the bowel, abdominal pain, wind, distension and (rarely) vomiting, may occur.

What can your doctor do?
- Your doctor will note the problems you are having and will take a family history, noting any relatives who have had bowel cancer and the age at which they developed it.
- Risk factors like smoking, obesity, lack of exercise may also indicate your susceptibility.
- He may suggest some tests. These may include a faecal occult blood test (FOB – a test which detects hidden blood in stools), blood tests (for anaemia and infection), and should also include a digital rectal examination (this means the doctor using a gloved finger).
- Women are sometimes given a pelvic examination, as 'bowel' symptoms can sometimes be caused by gynaecological problems.
- Preliminary tests may be followed up by a hospital visit for further tests (barium enemas, ultrasounds and x-rays, sigmoidoscopy or colonoscopy) and to see a consultant. A colonoscopy, where biopsies are taken for analysis, is the most accurate method of diagnosis.
- New tests for bowel cancer are constantly being developed. British cancer researchers are working on one that identifies abnormal colon cells from stool samples, which contain a protein called MCM2 – the test, which is less invasive and cheaper than colonoscopy, could eventually become an effective screening tool.
- If you tend to develop adenomas (perhaps through FAP), it may be advisable to have them removed periodically. These are not generally cancerous, but they may become so.
- Treatment: This depends on what stage the bowel cancer is found to be at when it is diagnosed. The doctor will try to determine – by feeling the tumour if possible, and using scans (like CT and MRI) – the size of the tumour and to what degree it has spread into its immediate surroundings. In addition, whole body scans can see if the tumour has spread to distant organs ('secondaries' or metastases). With this information, the doctor can then decide whether radiotherapy should be given before any surgery. Sometimes this is advised if

the tumour is extensive, as it can shrink it down to make surgery easier and more likely to succeed.

■ Surgery is the mainstay of treatment. Results do depend on the skill of the surgeon. Surgery involves removal of the area of diseased bowel, plus a section of healthy bowel on each side of the tumour and the surrounding lymph nodes. The removed section is always sent to the pathology laboratory for analysis.

■ Chemotherapy may be given after surgery. The value of chemotherapy is proven, although marginal. Chemotherapy is commonly given when the cancer affects the lymph nodes.

■ 5-FU/FA (5-fluorouracil and folinic acid) is a standard chemotherapy treatment given by intravenous injection, which has been used for over 40 years.

■ The above treatment has been largely superseded by more modern drug therapies including Campto (irinotecan) and Eloxatin (oxaliplatin), which are widely used in the US and Europe. In the UK, the National Institute for Clinical Excellence (NICE) has currently limited the use of irinotecan to second-line treatment rather than using it as a first-line measure, although trials using it (and other drugs) are being conducted.

■ Hair loss does not occur with chemotherapy for colorectal cancers because of the drugs used.

■ Follow-up: A recent study by Manchester researchers indicates that intensive follow up, which may include CT scans and frequent measures of serum carcinoembryonic antigen, improves survival rates.

■ Screening: A major UK study shows that routine screening for bowel cancer at the age of 60 offers a good, practical way to detect colorectal cancers, at early stages where treatment can be more successful.

■ Future developments: Scientists at Stanford University Medical Center are investigating the potential for a genetically engineered common cold virus to treat colon and gastrointestinal cancers that have spread to the liver. Early work indicates that the therapeutic adenovirus may be able to kill tumours without harming healthy liver cells.

What can you do?
■ Pay attention to your bowels. The key to spotting bowel cancer is noting a persistent change in your bowel habit that lasts more than two weeks. If this

occurs, always see your doctor, as bowel cancer often does not show any signs in the early stages.

- Look in the loo. Some people may think a visual inspection of what you've passed is disgusting, but it's a useful way to help you detect abnormalities like blood In the stool. It can also tell you if you're eating enough fibre – high-fibre stools are soft and thick, whereas low-fibre stools are heavier and tend to sink quickly.

- Don't be shy. Early detection of cancers significantly improves the chances of survival; so don't be too shy to seek help early. An audit of a Welsh hospital unit reveals that earliest stage cancer has an 80–90 per cent survival rate after 5 years, compared with 60 per cent for intermediate stage cancers, and less than 40 per cent for advanced cancers. A quick visit to your doctor gives you the opportunity to rule out any serious illnesses.

- Home kits are now available that can detect the presence of hidden ('occult') blood in the stools. They can show in a couple of minutes whether traces of blood are present.

- Evidence from Cancer Research UK suggests that regular exercise may halve your risk of bowel cancer. A daily half-hour of exercise is ideal.

- Lower the fat, raise the fibre. Studies confirm that eating more fibre (and eating at least five portions of fruit and vegetables daily) will reduce your risk of colorectal cancer. Whole grains may also have a protective effect.

- Avoid junk food. Dr Lesley Walker of Cancer Research UK says, 'High-calorie, meat-rich, low-fibre diets are likely to be contributory factors for bowel cancer.' She advises cutting down on high-sugar, high-fat, processed foods.

- Up the 'anti'. According to scientific research, antioxidants have powerful cancer-preventing properties. While most fruit and fresh vegetables contain them, the best candidates include blueberries, strawberries and raspberries. These contain large amounts of anthocyanins; ellagic, coumaric and ferulic acid (all phenols); calcium; and vitamins A, C, E and folic acid. All these are valuable anti-cancer and nutritive agents. Sweetcorn is an interesting exception to the rule that cooking may destroy some antioxidants – sweetcorn contains far more ferulic acid when cooked.

- Cut down your intake of animal fats and replace fatty cuts with lean meat. Avoid processed meats (they contain higher levels of nitrates) and salty meats like bacon and ham. Better still, replace red meat with chicken, fish and pulses. Avoid chargrilling food – it adds unwanted carcinogens to your diet.

- Take your vitamins. A recent study by the Dana–Farber Cancer Institute suggests that even people with a family history of colon cancer can significantly lower the risk of developing the disease by taking daily multivitamins that include folic acid (400 micrograms daily), and by limiting their alcohol intake to no more than two glasses of wine a day (or equivalent).
- Quit smoking. Smoking is causally related to all sorts of cancers – not just lung cancer.
- Maintain a healthy weight. If you're overweight, lose weight and keep it off.
- Know your family history. If bowel cancer runs in your family and you are offered screening, take it. Screening is also advisable for anyone with a pre-existing IBD, and for anyone over 50.
- See Self-Help for Bleeding (page 20), and Abdominal Pain (page 24).

Further information:
CancerBACUP, Telephone 0808 800 1234, and
www.cancerbacup.org.uk/info/colon.htm
Beating Bowel Cancer, www.beatingbowelcancer.org
Colon Cancer Concern, Helpline: 08708 506050 and www.coloncancer.org.uk

Stomach or Gastric Cancer

Stomach cancer occurs when a malignant growth develops in the lining of the stomach wall. There are several types of stomach cancer, but over 90 per cent are adenocarcinomas, which form tubular growths in the stomach and normally need treatment using surgery and chemotherapy.

What causes it? Scientists don't know the exact causes of stomach cancer, although they have identified several factors that can increase the risks of developing it.

- *Helicobacter pylori* infection is one of the prime risk factors for developing stomach cancer – experts suggest that it may play some part in up to 60 per cent of all gastric cancers.
- Stomach cancer is a particular problem in cultures where smoked, salted and preserved foods are widely eaten – like Japan and China.

Who can it affect?

- Stomach cancer is the second most prevalent cancer globally.
- It's twice as common in men than women.
- Roughly 25,000 people are diagnosed with stomach cancer in the US and about half this number die from it every year
- Of the 10,500 cases of stomach cancer in the UK each year, about 10 per cent run in families. Inherited forms normally strike early – in or before a person's 40s.

Age-bias: Stomach cancer is most common in the over-50s.

Risk factors:
- *H.pylori* infection
- Dietary risk factors include:
  - Smoked foods
  - High salt intake
  - Low intake of fresh fruit and vegetables
  - Pickled foods
  - High dietary intake of nitrates
  - High red meat intake, especially charcoal-grilled
- Smoking
- Excessive alcohol consumption
- People with blood type A are more at risk of stomach cancer.

Symptoms: The most common symptoms include:
- Weight loss
- New indigestion or heartburn (a burning sensation in the upper abdomen)
- Abdominal discomfort or pain
- Nausea and vomiting
- A new feeling of fullness or bloatedness after eating, although this is also a common symptom of IBS
- Difficulty swallowing ('dysphagia')
- A decrease in appetite
- Bleeding – either vomiting blood or 'coffee grounds' in the vomit

What can your doctor do?

- Your doctor will take a full medical and family history and may order some or all of the following tests:
  - Breath test for detecting *H. pylori*. If you test positive, you will normally be given antibiotics to clear the infection.
  - Faecal Occult Blood (FOB) test – to detect blood hidden in the stools, which may have come from the stomach.
  - Gastroscopy – which uses a flexible tube with camera that is swallowed by the patient under sedation or anaesthetic. This enables the physician to inspect the stomach more directly. Biopsies – tiny tissue samples – are taken for laboratory analysis. This is considered the best test for diagnosing gastric cancer.
  - Ultrasound scans – which can also show the condition of the stomach and upper GI tract.
  - Upper digestive tract x-rays using barium liquid (swallowed) are occasionally used.
- Treatment depends on the stage at which the cancer is detected, the type of cancer found, and factors such as the age and general health of the patient and the ability of the patient (or their desire) to tolerate certain therapies. Treatments include:
  - Surgery to remove the affected part of the stomach. This procedure is called gastrectomy.
  - Chemotherapy using anticancer drugs – in the hope of clearing up any remaining cancer cells. Chemotherapy is quite effective nowadays, although it is still more likely to be used to improve the patient's condition rather than cure the illness.
  - Radiation therapy using radiation focussed on the cancer site – this is only very occasionally used in the treatment of stomach cancer.

What can you do?

- Prevention:
  - Eat plenty of fresh fruit and vegetables.
  - Cut down on fat – long-term, the lower the fat content of your diet, the lower your risk of developing many cancers, including stomach cancer.
  - Limit your alcohol intake.

- Quit smoking – smoking may increase your risk of stomach cancer.
- Cut out salty, smoked and pickled foods. These methods of preserving food were popular before refrigeration, and are implicated in the development of gastric cancers. Avoid processed meats high in nitrates; smoked fish, meats and poultry; and avoid pickled food.
- Detection:
  - Most stomach cancers are diagnosed at a fairly advanced stage, which is why the 5-year survival rate for this cancer is as low as around 20 per cent.
  - Watch for symptoms. See your doctor if you are concerned, especially if there is a history of gastric or colon cancer in your family.
  - Scientists at Cambridge University believe that a very rare but inherited form of stomach cancer – hereditary diffuse gastric cancer (HDGC) – is directly linked to faults on the E-cadherin gene and that genetic screening could help susceptible families.
- See Self-Help for Nausea (page 17), Abdominal Pain (page 24), Diarrhoea (page 14), and Constipation (page 10).

Further information:
The Canadian *Helicobacter pylori* Website www.canadianhp.com
The American Cancer Society, www3.cancer.org
CancerBACUP, www.bacup.org.uk/info/stomach.htm

Anal Cancer

The anus is situated at the end of the rectum (which is the end portion of the large intestine). Its primary function is to allow faeces to pass out of the body whenever the rectum is full. Part of the anus is inside the body and part is just outside. The inner section of the anus is made of glandular tissue, whereas the outer part is essentially an extension of our skin. Between the inner and outer areas of the anus lies the anal margin, which contains two rings of anal sphincter muscles that close (or open) to control the expulsion of wind and faeces. Because the anus contains several different types of tissue, different forms of cancer may develop.

What causes it? The causes of this *rare* cancer are unknown, although scientists have reported links with the Human Papilloma Virus (HPV) infection and HIV.

Who can it affect? Anal cancer affects slightly more men than women – and homosexuals are a little more at risk.

Age-bias: The chances of contracting anal and rectal cancer increase (as with most cancers) with age.

Incidence: Very rare. According to the American Cancer Society, fewer than 4,000 new cases of anal cancer are diagnosed in the US annually. It accounts for about 1 per cent of large bowel tumours. The rate of anal cancer in men, particularly homosexual men, however, has increased.

Risk factors:
- According to several authorities, anal sex (and any activity which leaves your anus red, swollen and sore) increases your chances of developing anal cancer.
- Smoking
- Infection by the Human Papilloma Virus (HPV). HPV-16 is often identified in anal squamous cell cancers and there is evidence that HPVs also cause transitional cell (cloacogenic) cancers.

Symptoms:
- Bleeding from the anus
- Pain
- Itching or sensations of pressure around the anus
- Urgency and frequency of bowel movements
- Mucus discharge
- A lump in or near the anus

Always see your doctor if you have any of the above symptoms – in the vast majority of cases you will find your problems are caused by something much simpler and less sinister, like haemorrhoids, for example.

What can your doctor do?

- The outlook for any treatment of cancer is better the earlier the cancer is detected. Early stage anal cancer is normally treated surgically by excising the cancerous area.
- In many (and often in the more advanced) cases, chemoradiotherapy may be preferred so that the sphincter muscle that surrounds the anus can be saved, allowing you to pass waste as normal afterwards. See Chapter 18, Hospitals, Surgery and More ...

What can you do?

- Avoid STIs by using condoms. Always use a new condom when switching between vaginal and anal intercourse.
- Anyone engaging in anal intercourse should have an HPV test every one to three years.
- Stop smoking.
- Dietary help:
  - Avoid constipation – high-fibre diets are associated with lower risks of developing all varieties of digestive cancers.
  - Lower your dietary fat and make sure your intake of vitamin A is adequate.
  - Omega-3 fatty acids – these natural oils, found in flax seeds and oily fish (tuna, sardines, salmon), have a beneficial effect on the body. Flax seeds also contain anti-cancer antioxidants.
  - Other antioxidant-rich foods include tomatoes (a rich source of lycopene), blueberries and red grapes.
  - Nuts – Brazil nuts contain selenium, also believed to protect against cancer. Other nuts offer a wide variety of essential trace minerals (magnesium, manganese, phosphorus, zinc, copper), which help cells function healthily.
- See Self-Help for Bleeding (page 20), Itchy Bottom (page 31), Pain in the Back Passage (page 25), Urgency, Frequency and Incomplete Evacuation (page 29).

Further information:
Cancer Information and Support International,
www.cancer-info.com/analcanc.htm
CancerBACUP, www.bacup.org.uk/info/anal.htm

CHAPTER 17

Childhood Gut Problems

Children are prone to developing certain conditions already covered in other chapters – for example, constipation is very common among children, especially if there have been disruptions to their daily routine. Chronic constipation can cause minor, or superficial, anal fissures. Viral gastroenteritis often affects children, especially the winter vomiting viruses that can knock out virtually whole classrooms of school kids. Appendicitis is a common childhood emergency problem, and Crohn's disease and UC are not uncommon among older children and teenagers.

Where children tend to fare worse than adults is in their propensity for catching parasitic illnesses. The reason is fairly obvious: children are less aware of hygiene than adults and are forever putting things in their mouths that an adult might not – unwashed fingers and thumbs, toys found under bushes in the garden, even spiders, worms and other interesting nuggets! Children play outside, they stroke animals (often at the 'wrong' end) and come into physical contact with all sorts of bugs and germs. However, this is not altogether a bad thing – the 'hygiene hypothesis' suggests that living too sterile a childhood may create problems later on in life. The immune system can only function effectively if it is primed early in life to recognize the difference between 'me' and 'not-me' (i.e. foreign bodies, germs and viruses) – and it can't do this in too clean an environment. The increasing numbers of allergic conditions seen today indicate that perhaps there is not enough exposure to the natural environment early on in life. However, the hypothesis is not proven, and scientific research has thrown up conflicting opinions.

But the real problem for parents is not 'How can we protect our child from germs?' but more a case of 'How *much* exposure to germs will give them the maximum benefit for their developing immune system, without risking unnecessary or serious danger?' It's a question of degree ... and nobody knows the answer yet.

When our kids do get ill, another question that plagues parents is 'When do I call the doctor?' Infants and children are different from adults when they become unwell in one important way: they can become sick very rapidly, although they generally recover much faster as well. This makes time very much of the essence in paediatric medicine and every parent should always call their doctor sooner rather than later if there is anything that worries or concerns them about their child.

Always call your doctor immediately if:

- An infant has diarrhoea and vomiting that lasts more than 4–6 hours – dehydration can set in surprisingly quickly in babies and toddlers
- Your child has a high fever (temperature) – this can lead to convulsions if not brought under control
- There is abdominal pain, especially if it is accompanied by diarrhoea, constipation or vomiting
- Your baby or child goes unusually quiet, floppy, lethargic, drowsy (unable to rouse) or 'glassy-eyed'
- You are worried that your child may be suffering from a serious illness (like meningitis) – urgent treatment can prevent potentially fatal complications setting in

The good news is that mums (and dads) are normally equipped with a good gut instinct regarding their baby's welfare. We've all heard the stories about a parent's insistence that something was really wrong with their child leading to the child's life being saved. Use your intuition. You know your child best and you know when their behaviour or demeanour is not right. If you are concerned, always take your child to your doctor. It is far better to be labelled a worrier than it is to see your child on life support, and any doctor would rather examine a child unnecessarily than know that a parent didn't seek help soon enough.

Threadworm (Pinworm)

Threadworm (or pinworm) is a common childhood affliction and one that can easily spread through a family, especially among siblings who play together closely (and put their fingers in each other's mouths). The microscopic eggs of the parasitic worm *Enterobius vermicularis* can be found in house dust or contaminated food, and enter the body through the mouth. They travel through the host's digestive tract, hatch into worms in the small intestine and eventually emerge from the anus to lay their eggs on the surrounding skin at night. The tiny wriggling worms can cause intense itchiness. As a result, newly-laid eggs end up on the fingers and under the fingernails of an infected child, which, if put in the mouth, then start the cycle all over again. Threadworm infection is not considered dangerous, although it can disturb a child's sleep. In very rare cases, threadworm infection can cause appendicitis.

Who can it affect? Anyone, but children are especially susceptible.

Incidence: Threadworm is the most common parasitic roundworm infestation, affecting about one third of children in the US.

Age–bias: None known.

Risk factors:
- Poor personal hygiene
- Threadworm infections are slightly more common in warmer climates

Symptoms:
- Intense itching around the anus at night
- Soreness around the anus
- Possible mild abdominal pain
- Occasionally you can see the little white worms wriggling on the stools, or around the anus, at night

What can your doctor do?

- A swab, taken from the child's anus, can reveal the presence of threadworm eggs, although your doctor is more likely to ask you to look at your child's bottom at night with a torch (easier when they're asleep) – you can see the tiny white worms wriggling about around the anus as they emerge to lay their eggs.
- Your child will probably be given a dose of the anthelmintic drugs mebendazole or albendazole, the most commonly used drugs for threadworm infestation.
- The whole family should be treated as threadworms spread extremely easily between people, especially those in close contact.
- Treatment is normally repeated after two weeks to ensure that the infestation has been eradicated.

What can you do?

- Encourage your child to wash their hands properly and not to put their fingers in other children's mouths, or vice versa.
- Try to discourage scratching, as this can make the anus and surrounding skin very sore.
- Wash bed linen and nightclothes as they can be contaminated, and continue to change them regularly.
- Herbal help: Raw garlic is believed to be toxic to worms. A preparation of cayenne pepper and senna, mixed in a small amount of live yoghurt, is a herbal alternative to medicinal worm treatments.
- See Self-Help for Itchy Bottoms (page 31).

Further information:
Health Square, www.healthsquare.com/mc/fgmc0534.htm
Surgerydoor,
www.surgerydoor.co.uk/medical_conditions/Indices/T/threadworm_pinworm.htm

Encopresis

This frightening-sounding condition simply refers to children who start soiling their underwear after they have been previously (and apparently successfully) toilet-trained. It can be a response to an emotionally demanding situation, for example, moving house, a parental separation or divorce, or a new baby brother or sister. It can also be caused by chronic constipation. In this case, hard, dry faeces accumulate in the bowel, but loose, watery motions trickle past them out of the bowel.

Because toilet training is a somewhat hit-and-miss affair, accidents often happen. These are *not* encopresis. If they occur long after toilet training has successfully finished in a child over about 4 years of age, it might indicate the problem.

Who can it affect? Children. Boys seem to be affected much more often than girls.

Incidence: Encopresis is relatively common – accounting for an estimated 3 per cent of visits to paediatricians and 10–20 per cent of visits to paediatric gastroenterologists.

Age–bias: Soiling of this nature is only considered abnormal in children aged about four and over.

Risk factors: Stress is a risk factor. Things that are stressful for children may be different to those that are stressful for adults.

Symptoms:
- Diarrhoea or occasional soiling of underwear that may seem like diarrhoea
- A reason for emotional upset or disturbance
- Chronic constipation
- Occasionally the child may (either separately, or in addition) be found making bowel movements in odd places, like behind the sofa.

What can your doctor do?
- Your doctor may suggest a mild paediatric laxative or stool softener if severe constipation is a problem.
- If there are emotional issues involved, your doctor may refer you to a child psychologist or counsellor.

What can you do?

- You can help ease constipation by increasing the child's fibre intake (gradually) and liquid intake (quickly).
- If you suspect an emotional cause, don't punish, humiliate or embarrass your child. Instead, gently encourage him or her to uncover their anxiety.
- Go back over some of the basic toilet training routines and gently encourage your child to use the toilet at appropriate times – like after meals and before bedtime.
- Flower remedies: Rescue Remedy can help ease a child's distress.
- See Self-Help for Diarrhoea (page 14), and Constipation (page 10).

Further information:
Encopresis.org – www.encopresis.org

Intussusception

Intussusception occurs when a section of the intestine moves up inside another section of intestine, rather like a telescope. It not only causes severe abdominal pain, but can also cut off the blood supply to the telescoped section of intestine, leading to potentially fatal problems.

The cause remains unknown, although it is associated with enlarged intestinal lymph nodes following infections. Very rarely it may be caused by appendicitis or tumours. There is also a suspected (as yet unproven) connection with the tetravalent rotavirus vaccine (RotaShield®) that has been offered to infants in the US.

Who can it affect? Intussusception is the commonest abdominal emergency in infants aged between 3 months and 2 years, and is three times more common in boys than girls.

Incidence: Intussusception affects between one and four infants in every 1,000.

Age-bias: The peak incidence occurs in infants aged between 5–9 months, but it can also occur in newborns, older children and adults.

Risk factors:

- There is a slightly higher risk if it runs in the family
- Children diagnosed with cystic fibrosis who are dehydrated are at higher risk of developing it
- Children or infants with abdominal or intestinal tumours
- Children with gastroenteritis or an upper respiratory tract infection
- A handful of cases of intussusception were reported in the US within a few weeks after having been vaccinated against rotavirus. The rotavirus vaccination was withdrawn in July 1999 pending further evaluation. Rotavirus vaccination is not used in the UK.

Symptoms:

- Intermittent and severe abdominal pain, making the baby draw its legs up and cry
- Fever
- Stools resembling redcurrant jelly
- Vomiting
- Pale skin
- In between bouts of pain, the baby may be irritable or lethargic

What can you do?

- If you suspect intussusception, seek medical help immediately; surgery may be necessary.

What can your doctor do?

- If the doctor suspects intussusception he will arrange for the child to be admitted to hospital immediately.
- Your child will normally be given fluids intravenously and may have a tube put down their nose into the stomach, to prevent vomiting.
- Contrast x-rays using barium enemas are commonly used to definitively diagnose the problem. Because of the gentle pressure that the barium exerts inside the intestines, it often causes the telescoped intestine to pop out again, rectifying the problem. Sometimes air, rather than barium, is used.
- Surgery may be needed to relieve the obstruction, but recovery is usually quick and complete.
- Intussusception rarely happens more than once, and the outlook is very good.

Further information:

Kids Health For Parents,

www.kidshealth.org/parent/system/surgical/intussusception.html

American Academy of Paediatrics, www.aap.org/new/rotapublic.htm

Family Doctor, http://familydoctor.org/handouts/111.html

CHAPTER 18

Hospitals, Surgery and More ...

Now that we've examined what can go wrong with your guts, it is vital to take a look at what happens when we need hospital treatment or surgical intervention. Surgery is, for many illnesses, a last resort. It is not something that most of us will ever have to undergo. But it can happen and therefore needs to be discussed. People do occasionally need colostomies and ileostomies, and this book would not be complete if they weren't mentioned.

Hospitals

There are several reasons for hospital visits. They can be for minor tests at outpatient clinics, or planned admissions for more involved tests or for treatment, or even emergency admissions due to illness. They're all different.

The Outpatient Visit

This may be to see a consultant, or for minor tests. You will know exactly what you are there for, where it will happen and will be given any relevant information in advance – like whether you have to fast beforehand, or if you will need to give blood. Outpatient departments are normally the frontline department for the hospital (unless a patient comes in as an emergency). Outpatient clinics are often overbooked and very rarely run to schedule – so always take a good book or magazine to get you through a potentially long wait.

Inpatient Admission for Investigative Tests

This normally happens when you have a specific medical problem that needs further investigation, or if doctors need to do more involved tests that may, for example, require sedation or an anaesthetic, or so that doctors can run a battery of tests on you in one go. Normally, your stay will either be on a day-case basis, or you will be told how long they expect you to stay for – it's usually just a day or two.

Inpatient Admission for Treatment

The most common reason for an inpatient stay (other than for investigative tests) is for surgery. Sometimes the surgery is not vital, but is something the patient has chosen to have – as is the case with some hernias and perhaps haemorrhoids.

Surgery that is necessary (but not an emergency) is obviously planned in advance – for example, some patients with unresponsive UC or Crohn's disease may go into hospital for surgery when they are more or less in remission. This is often done because there is a better chance of surgical success when the patient is stronger, better able to withstand the physical demands of an operation and therefore able to recover quicker. Surgery is also more successful when the patient is either off or taking lower doses of steroids, as these drugs delay healing and need close monitoring after surgery. Polyp and tumour removal are another reason for a planned in-patient stay, although there is normally a greater degree of urgency in removing a tumour.

There are many things that you will wonder about before and during a hospital stay: write down your questions so you don't forget, and ask staff when they visit.

If you are having surgery, you will normally meet the surgeon at least once beforehand. Useful questions to ask include:

- How many of your particular operation have they done before, or how many do they do every month?
- What are the benefits of the surgery and what is the most likely outcome?
- What are the risks and are there alternatives?

- What were the outcomes of the most recent operations? The surgeon ought to know and you perhaps ought to be suspicious if they duck the question. If the surgeon gives figures to back his answer up, check that these are his own figures, not the national average.
- Is he part of a specialist team for your kind of operation? Cancer operations, for example, should ideally be done in a specialist or designated cancer unit.

Emergency Admissions

With emergency admissions there is generally little one can do! Emergency admissions may be due to peritonitis, severe gastrointestinal upsets like food poisoning, strangulated hernias, ruptured diverticula, intestinal blockages or many other reasons.

If you are admitted as an emergency, there is normally no time to think of anything – although paramedic staff may remind you to take house keys, a small toiletry bag, vital medicines, a change of clothes or pyjamas and slippers, and even a coat and some shoes. Remember, friends or relatives can always follow with any other items you need.

Tips for a Comfortable Hospital Stay

- Hospitals usually send a list of items you will need to bring; you can always ask for one if you need it.
- On admission you are normally given an information sheet or booklet explaining the daily routine, the staff that will help you and other useful bits of information.
- If there are things you want to bring from home to make you more comfortable, relaxed or better able to sleep, you can often bring them. Each hospital (and country) tends to have different rules, so ask beforehand about items like personal duvets and pillows, electrical equipment (for example, CD walkmans) and computers.
- Always remember to bring any normal medicines that you use. If you rely on hospitals to provide them, they have to be signed off by a doctor and this may take some time – an important consideration if your drugs have to be taken at precise times of day. Private hospitals generally charge for extra medication.

- Valuables and hospitals don't mix. There are few safe places to keep items like jewellery that you may have to remove before certain tests – so leave them at home.
- Toiletries are a must, so don't forget them – especially if you're fussy about what you use. Some hospitals do have a daily trolley service but this will usually only sell a limited range of toiletry essentials (as well as newspapers, snack foods and drinks).
- Nightclothes, a dressing gown and slippers, and a clean change of clothes for discharge are all good ideas. Socks can keep cold feet warm in hospital beds or while stuck on a trolley. Cardigans can keep your top half a bit warmer if you're sitting up in bed. Underwear is always a good idea to help preserve your modesty!
- Phone numbers and your diary can be useful – in case you need to rearrange any appointments or have to contact people in a hurry. Mobile phones are generally not allowed in hospitals, but there are often bedside phones or payphones.
- Unless you're on a restrictive diet, you will only get hospital meals at hospital times and you may be hungry or thirsty in between. You may be allowed drinks and snacks that don't need refrigerating.
- Hospitals are boring, especially when you're waiting for tests. Many provide TV and radio, but not when you're on a trolley in a corridor waiting for an x-ray! Take magazines, books or whatever whiles away those dull hours.

Being Stitched Up: Abdominal Surgery

There are many reasons for surgery – but the most common one is the removal of tissue – whether it is diseased through inflammation (due to UC or Crohn's disease, for example), or because of a tumour or growth.

Surgery can also be required to treat obstructions, repair fistulas or drain abscesses. Having removed any diseased tissue, surgery also often involves reconstruction, such as joining bowel together and/or creating an internal 'pouch' from the small intestine or colon to replace the rectum (if this has been removed).

What Normally Happens When You Have Surgery

- Once surgery is arranged, you may be given a date to attend the hospital for a pre-admission assessment. This appointment, often a week or two before the planned operation, gives the medical and nursing staff the chance to get to know you (and your body) beforehand. Chest x-rays, ECG and blood tests will be done and your blood pressure, weight, pulse and temperature will be taken. This gives the staff a base line measurement to use for future assessment, and it also gives them the chance to pick up any minor problems that might need resolving before your operation. This visit also offers you the chance to get to know the staff and ask as many questions as you like (regardless of how trivial they may seem).

- On admission to hospital, you will normally be visited by a member of the medical team, the specialist colorectal nurse and also the anaesthetist. Blood samples will be taken by a phlebotomist or venesectionist.

- After surgery, you may be in a Progressive Care Unit (PCU) or High Dependency Unit (HDU), depending on your medical needs. This is quite normal with abdominal surgery, especially if it is involved or lengthy. Food and drink (except sips of water) are normally withheld until the bowel starts working again. If you start drinking or eating too soon, there is a good chance that you will be sick.

- You will probably be attached to several tubes. IV drips are used to replace the fluids you are unable to drink and to allow medication (like antibiotics) into the bloodstream. Nasogastric tubes are often put down through your nostril into your stomach to prevent vomiting and allow any fluid that may collect in the stomach to be withdrawn. Urinary catheters are often inserted to allow medical staff to keep an eye on your kidney function and measure your fluid output. The good news is that this also spares you from journeys to the bathroom. You might also have a wound drainage tube in your abdomen to drain away excess fluid and blood that collects as a result of surgery.

- Major abdominal surgery usually requires a 10–14 day stay in hospital. More minor surgery (reversal of stomas, appendicectomies and so on) may only require you to be in hospital for 4–6 days.

Some Surgical Terms Explained

It's bad enough having surgery – but worse still when you can't even understand the jargon that you might hear (or overhear). Here are some key terms...

Anastomosis – the procedure of joining two ends of intestine together by stitching or stapling

Anterior resection – what happens when the diseased rectum is cut out and the remaining healthy ends are rejoined together, recreating the bowel as a continuous tube

Colectomy – removal of all or part of the colon, with the two remaining ends joined together afterwards

Colostomy – a stoma that is made using the colon

Ileostomy – a stoma that is made using the last part of the small intestine (the ileum)

Stoma – stoma is Greek for 'mouth'; a stoma is made when a section of the bowel (small or large) is brought out onto the surface of the skin in order to collect waste by affixing an appliance or bag onto the skin surrounding the stoma. A stoma can be permanent if the anal sphincter muscle has been removed. Sometimes a temporary stoma is given so that waste is prevented from passing through a healing join.

Total anorectal excision – this involves removing the rectum and anal sphincter muscle, and results in a permanent stoma (colostomy)

What Normally Happens after Abdominal Surgery?

Pain control: This can include any of the following:

- Epidural anaesthetic – where a spinal block is given to reduce or numb sensations from the abdomen downwards. Epidurals are normally allowed to wear off during the first few hours after surgery.
- Patient-Controlled Analgesia (PCA) – this allows the patient to control their own pain relief, within certain limits. This is normally done using a hand-held button, which can be pressed whenever pain relief is needed and which delivers a dose of an analgesic drug through the IV drip. The PCA system is designed so that the maximum amounts of pain medicine (as defined by the nurses and doctors) are not exceeded.
- Injections and tablets – these are normally given as pain starts to subside, 2–3 days after surgery, according to how the patient is coping. Some drugs (like pethidine), can make you feel sleepy or groggy, while others (paracetamol and related drugs) may not.

Mobilization Although moving about is generally the last thing on a patient's mind after abdominal surgery, starting to move is very important. It not only helps prevent chest infections from setting in (and is another reason why you may be slightly propped up in bed), but it helps prevent blood clots (thromboses) from forming.

Recovery of gut function As the gut recovers from surgery, first wind and then faeces will begin to emerge from the stoma or anus. As gut function returns, liquids are given by mouth – initially in small quantities, but later freely. Once liquids are being tolerated, a light diet can be introduced and at this point the IV drip can be removed (unless it is being used to deliver antibiotics or other drugs).

Removal of drains and urinary catheter Often, surgeons place a drain (a tube or piece of corrugated plastic) in the operation field, which is brought out onto the abdomen, in order to drain away any oozing blood. Drains are usually removed after 24–48 hours. It's also normal to have a urinary catheter, which is removed once the patient becomes mobile – usually between the

2nd and 6th days. Operations that are deep inside the pelvic cavity (near to the bladder and prostate gland) may cause difficulty in passing urine for a while – in which case a catheter may be left in a little longer. If a nasogastric tube has been placed through the nostril down into the stomach, it can normally be removed when the intestines start working again.

When Things Don't Quite Go According to Plan

Surgeons always do their best to avoid complications – but unfortunately they do occasionally happen...

Haemorrhage All operations incur a risk of bleeding (haemorrhage), although in fact this doesn't normally cause serious problems. Internal haemorrhages that are caused by the raw surfaces of intestine oozing blood often resolve spontaneously. Sometimes an internal blood clot or haematoma forms, which may need draining. Post-operatively, blood pressure and other vital signs are measured frequently. Signs of serious haemorrhage include a rapid, thready pulse, low blood pressure, pallor, dizziness, confusion and rapid shallow breathing. If serious haemorrhage is occurring, further surgery to stop the bleeding will be needed.

Infections
- Chest infections can cause a high temperature in the early days after surgery. An abdominal wound makes it painful to cough and phlegm may accumulate in the chest and become infected. Physiotherapy and antibiotics resolve this problem. You can help prevent chest infections by quitting smoking before an operation, getting as fit as possible and losing weight. After the operation, you can help by breathing deeply, trying to cough (while supporting the wound with a hand, a small pillow or folded towel), and by getting mobile quickly. Nurses will help you get up and about.
- Wound infections occur in 5–20 per cent of cases, depending on whether there was contamination in the abdomen – for example, due to an abscess or perforated bowel. When wounds become infected, they become painful and swollen and a fever will develop. Treatment includes draining the wound of blood and pus. The infection then usually settles and the defect in the wound will heal, although it may take a few weeks to completely close over.

- Urinary infections aren't common after intestinal surgery, but symptoms include burning sensations of passing urine, frequency of urination, lower backache and a fever. Treatment is with antibiotics.

Intra-abdominal abscess This usually occurs as a result of infection of a haematoma (see haemorrhage, above). It causes a fever and may slow the recovery of bowel function. A scan may be needed to locate it, and drainage may be necessary if it doesn't drain spontaneously. This can sometimes be done by inserting a fine needle through the skin (under local anaesthetic) into the abscess cavity – otherwise, surgical drainage under general anaesthetic will be necessary.

Thrombosis Surgery tends to make blood more liable to clot, which is why patients are almost routinely given regular injections of heparin (an anticoagulant) after surgery. Thrombosis (a blood clot) is most often seen in the veins of the leg or pelvis, and can result in swelling and pain, although not always. Diagnosis is made by clinical signs and by scans or x-rays of the veins (venograms). Treatment includes full anticoagulant drugs and close monitoring. Occasionally, a clot in the leg or pelvic vein may break away and travel up to the heart, where it can block (or significantly reduce) the blood outflow from the heart. This is a pulmonary embolism, a serious problem that may cause sudden collapse and even death, and which requires emergency treatment and resuscitation.

Intestinal Obstruction Surgery also causes the formation of adhesions (see page 123). Intestinal surfaces become inflamed and sticky and occasionally two sections of bowel may stick together, resulting in a kink or twist, which can lead to a partial or complete blockage (see page 183). If this happens, the abdomen will become distended or swollen, vomiting occurs and there is no bowel activity. Treatment usually involves emptying the stomach using a nasogastric tube, and giving water and electrolytes through an IV drip until the condition resolves (which it usually does). If not, or if there are fears that the blood supply to a section of gut may be completely cut off, surgery will be needed to straighten out the kink.

Breakdown of the surgical join (anastomosis) This is a serious complication that happens in about 5 per cent of cases where an anastomosis has been made. Faeces leak out from the intestine into the peritoneal cavity, causing infection. Symptoms include feeling ill, pain and a rapid pulse. The abdomen becomes swollen and tender, and the infection may cause general effects on the body like kidney, lung, liver and heart failure. Clotting mechanisms may also be disturbed. This condition has a significant mortality rate and urgent treatment – including IV fluids, antibiotics and more surgery – is needed.

Fistulation Sometimes when a leak occurs, faeces find their way out to the exterior without contaminating the peritoneal cavity. The discharge is usually through the wound or a drain site. If this happens, the patient is less ill than if the faeces stay inside the peritoneal cavity. The patient normally improves once the discharge or fistula has formed. Sometimes fistulae close on their own over several weeks but if not, surgical closure is eventually done. In the interim, parenteral nutrition (directly into a vein) may be given to prevent food from passing through the intestines.

Me and my Bag – Colostomies and Ileostomies

The words 'colostomy' and 'ileostomy' describe what to many people sound like drastic measures. In both cases they are necessary when a large chunk of intestine is removed, which also takes away the ability to empty the waste matter your body produces (faeces) in the normal way – i.e. out through your bottom. Having a colostomy or an ileostomy means that the waste comes out through a small, surgically-made hole on your tummy, to which a disposable plastic bag (or pouch) is attached.

So what's the difference between a colostomy and an ileostomy? Very little, other than to indicate at what point the opening – known as a stoma – is made. A *colostomy* is made when a section of the colon has been removed, including the rectum, anus and possibly anal sphincter muscles. The remaining end of colon is then made to empty out onto the abdominal surface. About 100,000 people in Britain have colostomies. An *ileostomy* is made when the entire colon has been removed, meaning that the ileum – the end of the small intestine – now has to empty directly out onto the abdominal surface. About 25,000 people in Britain have an ileostomy.

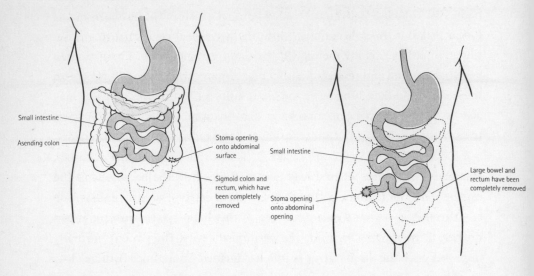

Colostomy (following removal of lower section
of large bowel and rectum)

Ileostomy (following removal of entire
large bowel and rectum)

Colostomies and ileostomies are not always permanent. Sometimes they are made so that internal stitching can heal following surgery. Very often, surgery involves cutting out a section of the intestine – perhaps where there is severe ulceration – and sewing the two healthy ends back together again. This is called 'anastomosis'. Temporary colostomies and ileostomies are often made to give the wound time to heal, and these are very easily reversed after a few weeks.

'Being told that I needed a colostomy was probably the most devastating news I've ever had. All I could focus on were the negative aspects – and I was convinced that my life would be severely limited afterwards. It never occurred to me that my life was already limited because of my illness. Getting back to normal has been difficult, and no one could have prepared me for the extent of the psychological "shake-up". But now 18 months later, life is good again. I'm comfortable with my appliance and now take it all in my stride. I've been abroad on holiday and have even started scuba diving again – something I never thought I'd be able to do with a bag attached to my belly.'

Martin, 46

Can You Eat Normally?

Because food has been completely digested by the time it reaches the colon, you are unlikely to need a special diet. The exception to this may be if you have had the terminal portion of your ileum (in the small intestine) removed, in which case you may need regular vitamin B12 injections.

Because the waste that travels through the small intestine is very watery, the output that comes from an ileostomy is always very liquid. With a colostomy, the output can be pretty thick – very similar to normal faeces. One of the biggest hurdles colostomists and ileostomists face is managing the output from the stoma. Because a stoma has no sphincter muscles, you can't control how often waste emerges and you also can't control any production of wind. Here are some tips:

- Too much fibre can cause excess wind – which can be noisy in a pouch and which can (if your pouch doesn't have a filter) cause it to balloon out. Typical windy foods include beans, peas, onions, leeks, grains, pulses and unripe bananas.
- Beer and fizzy drinks also increase the amount of wind you produce, are likely to make your output watery and can make your stoma very active!
- Foods which make wind smelly include fried onions, fish, cucumber and baked beans, but people differ and you'll normally be able to put together your own list soon enough.
- Chocolate and some fruit can also have a laxative effect.
- If your output is very liquid (as is the case with an ileostomy), certain foods may thicken it – marshmallows, ripe bananas, potatoes and pasta are good at decreasing pouch output. Bulking agents like Fybogel can be used to thicken the output. Cauliflower also helps some people, but can have the opposite effect in others.
- Certain foods and medicines can alter the colour of your output – for example, iron and charcoal (black), antibiotics (green), beetroot (red).
- Some foods are not broken down and will be passed whole, unless they are heavily chewed, mashed or puréed. These include mushrooms, peas and sweetcorn. Other foods like orange pith, unpeeled apples, nuts and celery are quite fibrous; sometimes it can feel as if the stoma is having difficulty pushing the waste through.

- Spicy foods can irritate the intestine and make you produce frequent, watery output. They can also irritate the stoma and surrounding skin (if there is any leakage).
- Ileostomists lose far more water in their waste than normal and therefore need to make sure they don't become dehydrated, especially in hot weather or during sport. Alcohol and caffeine are diuretics and may cause dehydration. Always drink more than the normal recommended amount of 2 litres per day. You may also need to increase your salt intake.

What about Sex?

An active sex life and an ostomy appliance are not mutually exclusive. True, there may be problems of self-image and practical considerations to overcome – but there is no reason why a sexual relationship cannot be as good, if not better (because you should no longer be ill), after a colostomy or ileostomy than it was before.

Surgery is physically exhausting and sex is not generally high on the priority list for many people during the earliest stages of recuperation. Nerve damage can occasionally leave a man temporarily or permanently impotent and, in this situation, a pump device or other sexual aids may help in restoring some degree of function (see page 242, which looks at male impotence). Stoma nurses are equipped to advise on this type of problem.

I'm a Kangaroo! Living with an Internal Pouch

When I was told that I was going to lose my entire large bowel, I automatically assumed I'd have a permanent ileostomy. That was, until my doctor told me about a special procedure called a 'total restorative proctocolectomy'. In a nutshell, it meant that I would still have my colon removed, but that a section of my small intestine would be refashioned to make a reservoir, or 'mini-colon'. The reservoir would then be reattached to my rectum and anus and – because the anal sphincter muscles would still be working – it would mean (barring a few subtle differences) that I could still go to the toilet as normal. I never realized until this point how important the ability to go to the toilet 'normally' was to me. I immediately signed up for one.

The procedure is not new. Sir Alan Parks developed the first ileo-anal pouches in the early 1950s. Admittedly, the techniques used then weren't quite as well honed (and as successful) as they are today, and yet it still strikes me as amazing that very few people seem to be aware of ileo-anal pouches even today, despite the fact that surgeons are increasingly offering them to patients. Many people still believe that extensive bowel surgery necessitates a permanent ostomy, when this isn't automatically true.

Internal pouches are quite tricky to construct and the procedure generally involves at least two operations rather than one. Not everyone's internal anatomy can be made to accommodate one. There are also higher risks of failure and post-surgical complication, and there hasn't been enough long-term experience with pouch-owners (in sufficient numbers) to know how long they can last for. There are also potential complications with infection, and they don't suit everyone.

How Are They Made?

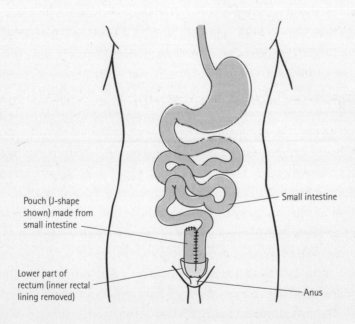

Pouch (J-shape shown) made from small intestine

Small intestine

Lower part of rectum (inner rectal lining removed)

Anus

The first stage of the procedure involves removing the colon – the colectomy. If this is done on its own, it is normally quite a straightforward operation, with the removal of the colon and formation of a temporary stoma. Recovery is generally very quick – about 8–10 days. Sometimes the colectomy and the formation of the pouch are done at the same time, in which case the operation is more lengthy and complicated, taking 4–5 hours (compared with about 1–2 hours for a simple colectomy). Pouches are made by looping the end of the small intestine into a 'J', 'S' or 'W' shape, and stitching it into place. ('W' pouches, which are more complex to make, offer the largest 'reservoir' capacity.) The pouch is then connected to the remaining end of the rectum. A temporary stoma is made, which allows the new ileo-anal pouch to heal properly before any waste is allowed to pass through it. After about eight weeks, the temporary stoma will be reversed and the pouch can start to work.

How Do They Work?

Very soon after surgery to remove a temporary stoma, the new pouch starts to work, although because the output is from the small intestine, what is produced is very watery (like diarrhoea). The frequency with which you may need the loo can also be high, especially at first. Sometimes, particularly at night when muscles are more relaxed, there may be some leakage. This can be a frustrating nuisance, but in most people it gradually subsides. About 80 per cent of patients are completely normal in this respect after the operation. Pads can be used and pelvic floor exercises are invaluable in helping strengthen the anal sphincter muscles.

Anti-diarrhoeal medication such as loperamide (Imodium) or codeine phosphate can be used to slow output and frequency. Most pouch owners tend to go several times during the day and once or maybe twice during the night. People do get used to this (women especially, who often need to pee several times a day anyway) and the best part is that urgency – that desperate need to dash to the loo – is rarely a problem.

Occasionally, the pouch may become infected, causing 'pouchitis'. Experts believe this may be caused by an overgrowth of certain bacteria in the pouch. The symptoms of pouchitis are actually very similar to those of UC – diarrhoea (more than normal), bleeding, increased frequency, sometimes urgency, generally feeling unwell and possibly a temperature. Treatment for pouchitis includes antibiotics, and occasionally steroids may need to be given. Studies are underway to investigate the value that probiotics may have in preventing and treating pouchitis and so far the results look promising, although much more research is needed.

the person behind
the illness

———

Our bodies, and how they work, affect every waking moment of our lives. And not just in a practical or physical way: illness can profoundly affect our moods and relationships. It can impact on our careers and financial security. It can alter our ability (or desire) to have children, our libido and sex life. This last section of the book looks at such considerations and how they impact on the person behind the illness.

And what about the future? Chapter 21 takes a closer look at probiotics, which doctors (and many other health practitioners) are increasingly viewing as one of the most promising leads we have for gut health.

CHAPTER 19

A Look at Depression

When the bottom falls out of your world because the world is falling out of your bottom

'I was so lucky on the face of it. I had a loving wife, a good job with a boss who knew about my illness because a relative of his had also suffered with it, and as much time off as I needed. I was young, with a great family and no serious money worries. It never occurred to me that I might have been depressed. I tried to banish all these negative thoughts from my head, but they wouldn't go. One day, I woke up and thought, "I'm losing it." I went to my doctor, who immediately recognized I was depressed. I was shocked by his diagnosis and yet I knew it made sense. It had been going on for over a year by this time.'

Derek, 39, who became depressed after discovering he had a chronic digestive problem

You've Just Been Diagnosed...

You've just been diagnosed with a gut problem. Perhaps you don't fully understand it, perhaps it sounds frightening, or perhaps it might involve restructuring your everyday life. It could be an ulcer, UC, Crohn's disease, a hernia, or even something that seems disastrous – like bowel cancer. Whatever it is, it's likely to throw you – even just for a moment.

People deal with news of this kind in different ways. Some people want to read every scrap of information available about the illness, while others try and ignore the problem, secretly hoping that it will go away if it's paid no attention. But of course that rarely happens and to compound matters there's another problem that can go hand-in-hand with chronic and debilitating illness – depression.

Twenty years ago, depression was a big taboo. People generally knew very little about it. Today, much of that ignorance persists – despite the fact that it is a common problem. Contrary to what many believe, depression is not usually characterized by a dramatic descent towards suicidal tendencies. It is usually more insidious, often creeping up upon the individual in a slow but relentless fashion.

What Can Cause Depression?

- **Illness** Feeling unwell, tired, in pain – all these things put us mentally on the back foot. Feeling down is a common problem for anyone who suffers with severe and /or chronic pain. Illness makes life harder to cope with. Problems seem bigger when we're unwell, and goals are harder to achieve. Even the fun aspects of life can appear very different – what might be a lovely and relaxing stroll in the park to a healthy person may simply be another tedious chore if we're unwell.

- **Problems with 'body image'** 'Body image' is a fundamental part of everyone's psyche. It represents how we feel about our bodies and what they mean to us. Generally, body image starts developing at a rudimentary level when we are infants, but it isn't fully established until we've been through puberty and reached adulthood. When our bodies let us down or fail, our body image is inevitably affected. Bowel problems, perhaps more than most illnesses, cause very embarrassing symptoms. Diarrhoea, wind, bleeding, incontinence – all of these are potential social nightmares that can cause problems with our body image, which can in turn lead to depression.

- **The destruction of the ego** Connected with the body image is the 'ego' – our secret self, which lies at the core of our personality. Just as bowel illnesses affect our body image, they can also affect how we feel as a person – how we rate our value to society, whether we think we are worth loving. Being chronically or seriously unwell can make us feel like a burden on those around us. We might question why our loved ones stick by us. We might worry that they will leave – for someone who's less hard work. We may worry that our colleagues will grow resentful of our frequent time off work, and that we could lose our job. We fear that our children will resent a parent who is always tired, or cannot run about playing football, or who is frequently in hospital and misses the nativity play or the school concert. Sometimes we start believing that perhaps we 'deserve' our illness – that it's because of something we've done in the past. All of these thoughts affect the ego and are common in people who have been diagnosed with a chronic or serious illness.

- **The destruction of the 'sexual self'** While bottoms are not primary sexual organs, many people find stimulation of the anus and rectum immensely pleasurable. Bottoms are very close to the sex organs and are strongly linked with sex. It's not uncommon for a bowel problem to interfere with your sex life and how you see yourself sexually. Practical problems can interfere: administering an enema last thing at night may hamper the ability or desire to have sex. Having a fissure, or a tender stomach, or pain, can interfere with your ability to have penetrative sex. Having constant diarrhoea or incontinence can destroy your image of yourself as a sexually desirable person and make you feel worthless. Having a stoma may affect a man's ability to sustain a satisfactory erection and achieve ejaculation.

- **Practical problems** When a person with active UC or Crohn's disease goes shopping, they usually plan their route meticulously. They know where all the public toilets are, they know which shops accept their 'Can't Wait' card, and may carry a spare pair of underpants, wet wipes and tissues 'just in case'. Because of these illnesses (which cause frequent and often uncontrollable diarrhoea), they need to be prepared – or face the consequences. But it's mentally draining to always be 'on guard'. Having limitations on your social life can be depressing – not being able to spend an afternoon picnicking in the countryside because you'll need the loo, not being able to join in certain sporting activities, or knowing that you can't wear a bikini because your ostomy appliance may show – all these (and more) may contribute to feeling low.

- **Uncertainty** Some illnesses have a well defined onset, progression and outcome – for example, haemorrhoids that develop during pregnancy are usually quite easily treated and, although they can recur, they don't normally lead to anything more serious. If your appendix becomes inflamed it will be removed and, in the vast majority of cases, that is the end of the matter. But some illnesses – most typically UC and Crohn's disease, but also IBS, polyps and some cases of diverticulosis – have neither a clear pattern of progression nor a clearly-recognized outcome. You can have one severe attack of colitis and never suffer another. You can have mild bouts of colitis for 30, 40 or 50 years, where your disease never worsens. You can start with mild colitis located in the rectum (proctitis) that gradually worsens and spreads along the entire colon in a matter of years, or you can have a sudden, serious attack that destroys your entire colon in a matter of weeks. When there is no pattern, life can be tougher. Although we are naturally resilient, we don't like surprises. We want consistency and predictability. Illnesses that flare up unexpectedly are tougher to cope with because they are harder to predict and plan for. Is my diarrhoea going to be a problem on my best friend's wedding day? Is my illness going to flare up while I'm on holiday – and if it does, will I be able to find medical help? Problems make us feel helpless. And helplessness can contribute towards depression.

How Do You Recognize Depression?

Depression can be tricky to recognize – even in yourself. Sometimes it can come on suddenly – like the classic 'baby blues' that affect new mothers. But depression may not happen with a dramatic and recognizable bang. It can creep up insidiously, until you are engulfed by it – I call it 'stealth depression'. Because people are instinctive copers, they acclimatize to increasing depression as it grows and may not even be aware that things have subtly but significantly changed.

There are some classic signs of depression that anyone with chronic illness should know about. It helps if your partner and your family know too. The following list includes some of the more common signs of depression:

- Lack of energy
- Difficulty sleeping – especially waking very early in the morning
- Low self-esteem
- Feelings of anxiety and doom
- Feelings of hopelessness and worthlessness
- Difficulty concentrating and making decisions
- A loss of libido
- Lack of interest in food, or possibly eating more than normal ('comfort eating')
- Suicidal thoughts. Almost all people suffering from mild to moderate depression do not entertain suicidal thoughts. **If you experience suicidal**

thoughts or want to harm or kill yourself, seek help immediately. Samaritan groups or emergency medical facilities can be contacted 24 hours a day.
The Samaritans, Tel: 08457 90 90 90 (UK) or 1850 60 90 90 (ROI).
www.samaritans.co.uk

Then Again, You May Not Have Depression...

'I was so frustrated. I felt tired, I had chronic diarrhoea, my stomach hurt and I couldn't get a diagnosis. My doctor told me I was depressed and wanted me to start taking antidepressants. I didn't want to. I knew I wasn't "depressed" – I was bloody fed up though, because I couldn't go out anywhere and I couldn't find out what my problem was!'

Carol, 44, who suffered not from depression, but from an unsympathetic doctor

Many people – especially those with IBS or adhesions – are often told that a problem is 'all in their mind'. And although stress and unresolved emotional issues may cause or trigger conditions like IBS, nobody likes being called a hypochondriac.

Feeling unwell, especially over a long period of time, can cause unhappiness. This doesn't automatically mean we have clinical depression. Admittedly, some people do live in denial of depression but equally, others are sometimes accused of having depression when perhaps they don't and are physically suffering more than anyone recognizes.

What's the answer? Is there a trick? Possibly. The first thing is to be honest with yourself. Think carefully about how you feel and why you believe you feel that way. If you are reasonably self-aware, the answer may become obvious. You may decide that your mood is a direct result of your illness. On the other hand, there may be something that you can't explain, or that you recognize as 'not normal' for you – and if any feelings start to overwhelm you with their strength or persistence (for example, urges to harm yourself or desperate feelings of unhappiness) then seek help immediately. One person I know said, 'I only knew what depression felt like because I had post-natal depression after the birth of my first child – I would never have recognized it otherwise.'

How to Cope with Depression

There are several useful techniques for combating depression:

- **Exercise:** Regular exercise encourages our body to release endorphins – natural feel-good hormones that act as painkillers and lift your mood. If you're very unwell the type or amount of exercise you can take may be limited, but even a walk outside can help. Exercise is a great tonic for the soul and the body.
- **Herbal help:** St John's wort is very popular as 'Nature's Prozac' and has been used for hundreds of years to help relieve anxiety and depression. Sunbathing or sun exposure should be avoided while using it, as it can cause skin sensitivity. It may also cause allergic reactions in hypersensitive individuals, and should be avoided during pregnancy and breastfeeding.
- **Medication:** Many antidepressant drugs are available, most of which work by keeping serotonin and norepinephrene levels higher by stopping these important mood chemicals from being reabsorbed by brain cells. They include:
  - Selective Serotonin Reuptake Inhibitors (SSRIs) – This group of commonly used drugs for depression includes fluoxetine (Prozac), fluvoxamine (Luvox, Faverin), citalopram (Cipramil, Celexa), paroxetine (Seroxat, Paxil) and sertraline (Zoloft, Lustral)
  - Tricyclic antidepressants – This group includes amitriptyline (Domical, Elavil) clomipramine (Anfranil) and imipramine (Tofranil)
  - MAOIs – These include moclobemide (Manerix), phenelzine (Nardil) and tranylcypromine (Parnate)
- Dietary tips:
  - Peanuts, almonds, soybeans, sesame seeds, cheese and other protein foods contain the natural chemical L-phenylalanine, believed to help alleviate bouts of depression. Other amino acids (including L-glutamine, DL-phenylalanine and L-tryptophan) offer similar effects. Avoid amino acid supplements if you have been prescribed MAOI antidepressants, if you have high blood pressure, or if you are pregnant or breastfeeding.
  - Foods rich in B vitamins, like oats, cereals and whole grains, nuts and green vegetables, can help relieve depression and stress.
  - Clove tea can help raise the spirits.

- Flower remedies: Gentian helps encourage a positive attitude and may alleviate mild depression and despondency, while mustard is used for more severe depression. Rescue Remedy can help restore calmness during stressful situations.
- Aromatherapy: Most of the citrus oils – grapefruit, neroli (orange blossom), lemon, mandarin and citronella are uplifting and help relieve depression and mental stress. Herbs with anti-depressant actions include jasmine, basil, geranium, patchouli, clary sage and thyme. They can be used in aromatherapy massage and several may also be eaten as foods (citrus fruit, basil and thyme).
- Homoeopathy: Remedies used to alleviate depression include gold (*Aurum metallicum*), witch hazel (*Hamamelis virginiana*), ignatia amara, rock salt (*Natrum muriaticum*) and wind flower (*Pulsatilla*).
- Counselling and psychotherapy: A problem shared is a problem halved – talking through problems can relieve depression and stress. Qualified counsellors are available for those suffering from depression (though there may be a waiting list and you may need to press your case), anyone undergoing major surgery, who may have to have a stoma, or who may be incontinent as a result of illness.

Further Information:
Depression Alliance, www.depressionalliance.org/
National Foundation for Depressive Illness, Inc., www.depression.org/

CHAPTER 20

Coping

Coping with Flare-ups: Living a Normal Life

Any illness that flares up from time to time brings a series of unique problems. One is predictability – or the lack thereof. Whether you're planning a holiday or just a shopping trip, you naturally want it to coincide with a good patch rather than a bad one. However, the nature of flare-ups means you can't predict your health very far in advance, so you might need to start living more spontaneously.

Flare-ups interfere with virtually every area of life. Work can be disrupted, social events, outings with your kids – even doing the grocery shopping. Everything is a completely different ballgame when you're battling against a recurring illness. What you have to do is develop flexible coping strategies for dealing with flare-ups. Here's how...

Become Two People

Think of yourself as two people – one who is well and one who is slightly more disadvantaged (because of your illness). When organizing your daily life, always let the 'well' person make the plans. Then assume it may be the unwell person that is on duty on any given day.

Friends are generally understanding if you tell them in advance what your limitations might be, depending on how well you are that day. Let's look at an example. You and a friend want to meet for an all-day shopping trip. Plan it, but explain that if you are feeling below par you may only be able to come for a short shopping session, or maybe meet just for lunch, or you might have to cancel completely. Tell them you will let them know nearer (or even on) the day. Genuine friends won't have a problem with this; if they do, or they can't see things from your point of view, you may want to reassess the friendship.

Should I Go on Holiday?

Holidays, trips and treats are the food our souls live on. We all need breaks, whether we're confined to a wheelchair, using an artificial voice box or fighting another course of steroids. The increasing ease (and decreasing cost) of travel means that holidays and trips are more of a right than a luxury these days. And – perhaps *especially* when you have a chronic illness – you need outings and vacations to look forward to.

Plan for the Best, Prepare for the Worst

Whenever you commit yourself in advance to anything, use this strategy to help you. It's based on the Minimax principle – which means *mini*mizing your *max*imum loss.

- With travel, always take out insurance in case you are not well enough to travel on the day. Many travel policies exclude pre-existing conditions. Check with your local support group – they generally know specialist Insurers who will cover your condition.
- When you make plans – and this includes packing your suitcase – assume that you will be well and able to engage in whatever activities you had planned (so take your tennis racket, scuba gear or rock climbing equipment), but prepare for the fact that you may become ill while away.
- Always take the following with you:
  - Any medication you need when you are ill, in sufficient quantity to cover your whole stay. Travel with (at least) some of it in your hand luggage in case your luggage gets lost. You may need a letter (to show customs officials) explaining that you need the drugs for medical reasons.
  - 'Everyday' medicines and non-prescription items that you use – for example, bulking agents like Fybogel, anti-diarrhoeal medicines, anti-spasmodic drugs and vitamin supplements.

- A letter, clearly explaining your problem, that can be given to any medical personnel should you need treatment, especially if there is a language barrier. It's useful to find out what your condition is called in the language of the country you are visiting, in case you need to tell someone about it.
- Medicalert talismans (or a steroid card) are important if you are taking medication that should not be stopped suddenly, if you have a serious allergy (for example, to penicillin), or if you have a condition that doctors must know about before giving emergency treatment.
- A valid prescription for your key medicines.
- British citizens should carry an E111 – this medical form entitles British citizens to reciprocal healthcare within EU nations.
- Valid medical insurance cover, especially if you're travelling to places where private healthcare is the only option.
- Contact telephone numbers of your specialists, consultant and doctor for emergency use.
- Credit card to pay for emergency healthcare if needed (sometimes you may have to pay first and be reimbursed later by your insurer).

Of course you will have more luggage, you will have to be organized and think ahead, but you will also enjoy yourself and relax much more knowing that you are prepared for every eventuality. And that's important.

Coping with Strange Reactions

People say the funniest things. Some are intentional; others aren't. People often and quite easily put their foot in it by using the wrong words. 'What a bummer', 'You must feel like shit', 'At least it's all behind you now', 'It's such a pain in the arse' – all these, and more, can easily pop out of a friend's mouth, or your own. Learn to recognize when someone is simply using an unfortunate turn of phrase and treat it exactly as you ought to – with humour. Sometimes these inadvertent comments can lighten up what is often a tricky, uncomfortable or embarrassing moment. If it can be turned into a joke, enjoy it. After all, everyone has a skeleton in their closet. You may as well make yours dance.

Being in a Low-tolerance Zone

It's often when you're ill and don't feel like coping with all the extra crap that life brings, that people come out of the woodwork and make you feel even more miserable.

'Whenever I was unwell and on steroids, people would see my face all full and round and red, and tell me how well I looked. I often looked better when I was ill, because with steroids I'd gain a little weight, instead of being razor-thin. I used to get really fed up with people not understanding how my illness worked.'

Charles, 26, who suffers from Crohn's disease

Luckily, Charles discovered an obvious but useful little trick in dealing with it. He reminded himself that although he was hearing the same tedious and annoying comment for the umpteenth time, this was the first time that the person he was speaking to had made it, and that everyone was allowed at least one 'strike'. He also found he could also respond by smiling broadly and saying, 'Thanks. You should see me when I'm really well … I look even better then!' It was enough to get them off his back, without offending them, and would normally end the enquiries about his well-being.

Remember – when we're unwell, in pain or worried, we can also have a short fuse. Make sure that you're not taking your illness out on those around you.

Finding Mutual Support

Think of an illness or problem and you can bet your bottom dollar that out there somewhere is a support group for it. It's a testament to human nature that people who suffer from some of the most hideous problems still find the time, energy and generosity to help others in the same situation. Some people dismiss support groups, saying that they just encourage people to moan about their problems. Not so. Support groups provide a real link for people who might otherwise feel totally isolated because of a situation or illness that they never chose to have, and have no control over.

You don't have to be gregarious or extroverted to get something out of a support group. Many people find it enough simply to read a quarterly newsletter and pick up a few tips, in the comfortable knowledge that they are not alone. Others enjoy meeting other souls who truly 'know how it feels' and develop close and lasting relationships with them. You can be as involved as you want to be. Good groups encourage participation without coercion and offer people the services they want and need. They can also offer information that might otherwise be hard to come by: insurance tips, breaking medical news, conferences, access to drug trials and more.

Coping with Ignorance

Some people are surprisingly ignorant about health. They may have rarely been ill themselves, or may have absolutely no interest in medicine and their bodies. They may shy away from medicine because of deep-seated fears that if they acknowledge disease, they might somehow become more susceptible to it.

And because of the embarrassment and taboos surrounding bowel illnesses, people don't talk about them openly and often, which may add to your problem. Not everyone will automatically know about your illness when you mention it. And when they do, it's often because of a personal link. A typical response to hearing you have diverticulitis might be 'Oh, I know about that, because my aunt/mother/grandpa/best friend has that.'

Some people don't like to admit they're ignorant about your illness, while others may react by giving you a Spanish Inquisition – at a time when you might not feel up to all the questions. When I was suffering with UC, with three young children and a husband who travelled constantly and worked long hours, I often relied on the goodwill of friends to help me out. But I also felt uneasy about asking for help without telling them *why* I needed it. This meant explaining about my illness. During an active phase of disease, I would often have to dash to the loo *up to 14 times* before 8 a.m. My guts would quieten down during the middle of the day and I could often manage shopping and household chores before they 'activated' again later on in the day, leaving me washed-out and exhausted.

I wanted to explain to my friends why they might see me busily doing grocery shopping at 11 a.m., when at 8 a.m. I was apparently incapable of leaving the house. It's not always clear to people that illness can be like that. Sometimes I was happy to be single-handedly educating everyone I knew, yet at other times I really didn't want to have to explain a damned thing. I was too tired. But I also knew that as long as people kept quiet, the ignorance would persist. So I kept on explaining.

Other people don't feel as I do, and may not feel inclined or obliged to explain anything – there is no right or wrong way to go about it. If you don't want to explain, you don't have to. You can always dodge the question or give a vague answer. Do what feels right for you.

Coping with Rudeness and Unhelpfulness

Rudeness and unhelpfulness happen all the time, whether it's someone stealing the parking space you've been patiently waiting for, or pushing in front of you in a queue. But it feels worse when we're unwell or have special needs.

Many people with bowel problems need the toilet urgently and in such circumstances a 'Can't Wait' card is always useful. It can help if you're in a situation where you might encounter unhelpfulness – like when you're stuck on a plane and the stewardess tries to stop you going to the loo because the seatbelt signs are on.

Sometimes people simply refuse to budge, or make hurtful comments. There's no easy answer, but here are some tips that may help:

- Always try to show some kind of evidence, like a NACC 'Can't Wait' card. This often helps smooth a quick path to the loo and can also diffuse potentially unpleasant situations before they start.
- If this fails, explain politely what you need (there may not always be time) and the reason for your urgency.
- Try someone else if the person you've approached is being unhelpful (time permitting).
- Always try to stay calm, and avoid swearing/abuse at all costs. You automatically lose credibility and sympathy if you start cussing at people.
- If you do experience an embarrassing disaster as a result of someone's refusal to allow you access to toilet facilities, before you leave the scene, make sure you take a note of the person's name or at least a physical description. Write a strong letter of complaint to the manager/head of any authority or

company, detailing exactly what happened. Rude people often only learn the error of their ways when their unpleasantness comes back to haunt them.

- Sometimes, people are rude because they just are. You can't do anything about them, so don't take it personally.

Coping with a Partner: Sexuality and the Passion Killers

Gastric conditions such as wind or diarrhoea don't normally bring out the romantic side in us, and digestive problems can profoundly affect personal relationships and sexual activity. Making love is as much a mental act as a physical one and when our feelings toward our partners or ourselves are disturbed, our sexual relationships are inevitably affected.

'She thought I was rejecting her, but the truth is, I was scared of hurting her. After all, there had been a lot of reconstructive handiwork in that area of her body. It ultimately didn't matter how often I reassured her: she didn't believe me and thought I didn't love her or find her attractive any more.'

Jim, aged 46, talking about his relationship with partner Sally, who underwent a total restorative proctocolectomy after suffering with UC

Fear can affect a sexual relationship and in Jim's case, his fear of hurting Sally means that he is reluctant to have sex with her. Sally, in turn, is taking Jim's lack of sexual advances to mean that he no longer finds her sexually desirable. Tracey Virgin-Elliston, Stoma Care Nurse Specialist at London's West Middlesex University Hospital says, 'It is very common for partners to worry that they might hurt or damage the patient if they engage in close physical contact – like cuddles and sexual intercourse. The patient can then feel they are not desirable any more, especially if they have a stoma.' Self-confidence also plays an important role in sexual relationships. If we feel unattractive we also feel unsexy. In fact, Sally's desire for sex may well have increased after her operation, as she would be feeling much better than when she was chronically ill. Both partners need reassurance. 'Nurse specialists will see partners together and encourage intimacy,' says Tracey. 'In my experience it's never a good idea to start sleeping in separate beds after the patient leaves hospital unless they have always slept apart. It is very difficult to get back to the stage of sharing a bed, and the intimacy can be difficult to recapture.'

'I feel so unsexy because of my IBS. I feel stupid trying to be all glam and vampy knowing that any minute I'll have to rush to the bathroom, blasting wind and diarrhoea – all within earshot of my lover. How can any woman feel attractive and sexy when they're like that? It's ridiculous. I've given up dating because I feel so unsexy.'
Joanna, aged 22

Joanna is one of many hundreds of thousands of young adults affected by bowel problems. She should be enjoying her youth, her body and her relationships. Her IBS has taken away her confidence to do this – as she quite rightly says, it can be tough feeling feminine and attractive when your guts are misbehaving. Her IBS has meant that she's retreated out of the dating scene – a very common reaction for anyone suffering with gut problems. But it can work. The answer is to be upfront and honest with your partner – after all, farting is something we all do, even if it's with less gusto or not as frequently. 'A sense of humour is vital, and a loud stereo doesn't hurt, either,' advises Tracey Virgin-Elliston.

And dating needn't be a disaster, as single mum Amanda, aged 26, found out...

'Because of UC I recently had an ileostomy. It was hard for me to feel attractive and sexy at first, but I overcame the image problem by wearing the right clothes. Being a single mum, I don't get out much to date, but I did by chance meet a man recently. Once we got to know each other a little, I told him all about my operation and it didn't bother him. I was worried about the intimate stuff – what would happen when he saw "it", whether it would get in the way or make horrible noises – well, I needn't have worried because everything was great! I forgot it was there and we both got used to it. He said he was going out with me – not my bag...'

Occasionally, nerve damage during surgery interferes with a man's ability to achieve erection and ejaculation, and may also interfere with fertility (of both sexes). But even if there is no permanent legacy, surgery is still physically demanding and for several weeks afterwards you may simply not have the strength or stamina to perform as you might like.

'I couldn't achieve an erection after I had my colostomy – and when I did manage one, it was too short-lived to do anything much with. It was totally devastating.'

Gordon, aged 56

Tracey Virgin-Elliston explains, 'A high proportion of patients – depending on factors like the site of the surgery – will suffer from sexual dysfunction following major bowel surgery, especially when their bottom is sewn up and a permanent colostomy or ileostomy is made. This is due to damage of the nerves that cause erection or ejaculation. Any patient that this may happen to will have discussed it at length with their consultant and/or nurse specialist before the operation. Often function does come back with time, but if dysfunction persists after about six months, follow-up help will be given. Treatments include oral medication like Viagra, alprostadil, a drug that can either be given as a small pellet that is inserted into the tip of the penis e.g. MUSE, or by an injection into the base of the penis e.g. Caverject. There are also aids like vacuum pumps and penile implants that can help you achieve and maintain an erection. Stoma nurses can tell you about the wide range of techniques and equipment that can help.'

Of course, not all sexual dysfunction is physical. There are many psychological reasons for failing to achieve and sustain erections – like altered body image, performance anxieties and so on. It is important to give it time and to talk to your partner. Don't expect to be back to your old level of performance immediately. Remember that non-sexual physical affection can be as important as full-on sex, so take your time and enjoy massaging each other, or simply cuddle, stroke and reassure each other. If extra stimulation is what you need and reading sexy material together does it for you, then go ahead. Things generally get better if you don't berate yourself and you retain your sense of humour.

Sexual activities are always more comfortable if an ostomy appliance is emptied beforehand (and there is less risk of it coming off). A little tape can prevent an ostomy bag from flapping about or getting in the way. Avoid alcohol before sex, because it makes the output very liquid. Try not to knock or bump your stoma – they do tend to bleed easily. A little experimentation with positions will help (and may even increase your repertoire).

'Trying to be passionate when your partner is chronically unwell is not easy. Jane is always tired and has little enthusiasm for sex. If she isn't tired, she is in pain, or rushing to the bathroom, or having retention enemas. I try so hard to be understanding and supportive, but I am equally very frustrated because my sexual needs are not being met.'

Tim, aged 35

Being chronically and seriously unwell can affect many things – sex included. Jane's illness – including her nightly retention enemas – are getting in the way of Tim's sexual needs and while his problems need addressing, so do Jane's. When you're unwell you can be too tired to make love, or it may be physically uncomfortable. Some people may think Tim is being selfish wanting sex while Jane is chronically ill; however, unfulfilled sexual urges are tough to handle on a long-term basis. Jane and Tim have to meet somewhere in the middle if they want to keep their relationship strong.

When this type of problem arises, a little restructuring can go a long way. Make sure you face your partner when you give yourself an enema (you have to lie on your left side to do them). Eye contact, the ability to talk and even cuddle helps people feel close. Another way of getting round the practical problems of medication is to make love at other times of day, or have sex just before a nightly enema. If one partner has little interest in penetrative sex, they could think of ways to give the other sexual satisfaction – for example using oral or manual sex.

'I cannot explain why, and know I ought to feel badly about what I did, but our relationship was still quite new when he became ill. I just didn't fancy him any more, even though I tried to make myself, and eventually I had to leave.'

Susan, aged 34

Normally we would hear this problem from the perspective of the abandoned partner, but I specifically picked Susan's point of view because I don't believe that any situation is ever as clear-cut as we'd like to think. Relationships do fail during or after a crisis and for a million different reasons. But often the relationship was already doomed and the illness may just offer a good excuse for leaving.

So what do you do if your partner abandons you after a serious bout of illness or major surgery? It does happen. How do you cope? First, no matter what they may blame it on, realize that the outcome would have eventually been the same even if you'd never been ill. And if you really feel that they left you because (and only because) of your scar/ostomy/adhesions, then also realize that it's their loss and not yours.

Let's go back to Susan's comment that she 'just didn't fancy' her boyfriend anymore, even though she tried to. Sometimes when we see a person after major surgery, we may feel shocked by their appearance. Seeing our partner with a bright red stoma sticking out of their belly can elicit a variety of reactions ranging from fear and disgust to sadness and even anger. Usually, it takes a little while to get used to the change, but after a few days or weeks we realize this is the same person we knew all along. Counselling or talking to a stoma nurse can help enormously, as can talking with your partner and discussing your feelings together. They are probably just as disgusted/frightened/sad as you are.

In most cases, people who have had stomas or abdominal surgery confirm that their relationships usually grow stronger as a result. But it is equally possible, especially when two people are still learning about each other, that shattered perceptions and images of people fatally injure a budding relationship. Susan's image of her partner may have been destroyed by his illness. Although the definition of what makes someone sexually attractive may differ from one person to the next, it does underpin most successful relationships. The chances are that even if her boyfriend had never become ill, Susan would have eventually realized he wasn't right for her anyway.

Summary
- Reassurance and confidence are two key factors that underpin sexual success and happiness. They can both be achieved by talking to others in similar situations and by communicating with your partner in an open and loving way.
- Trying different techniques and methods can solve many sexual problems, whether they are physical or psychological.
- There must always be give and take; it is the responsibility of both partners to focus on each other's needs.

- When a partner is physically altered by surgery, it may take a little time to get used to the changes. It is quite normal for both partners to be upset or shocked at first, but this usually passes.
- Relationships break down constantly. Don't let anyone blame your illness for the break-up; instead realize that it would probably not have worked out anyway – people often use illness (or its consequences) as an excuse.
- Don't let a partner's illness hold you in a relationship that isn't working. If you realize you need to end the relationship, do it tactfully and with good timing (i.e. not when they've just come out of hospital).

CHAPTER 21

The Future for Gut Health

If I Had a Crystal Ball ...

There are hundreds of millions of pounds and dollars being spent on research into digestive illnesses. Virtually every day there is a news snippet suggesting that either a new drug is on the horizon that may cure a certain gastric disease, or that a dietary supplement shows promise in healing or preventing certain gut disorders, or that a gene is close to being identified that may partly explain some people's apparent susceptibility to developing certain digestive illnesses.

It is impossible to know which of these will ultimately prove true, especially as scientific advances are often reported to the public in their earliest infancy, several years before they may (or may not, in many cases) become a reality. And by the time any new drug hits the market, or the gene is isolated, there is usually even more research coming through which makes it look old hat.

The one thing that I have been struck by in the course of writing this book is not how many things can go wrong with our guts, but how incredible it is that they work so well. Nature has made our bodies so perfectly that even the best medicine and the most skilled surgery all tends to look amateur in its effort to put things right.

Nature is incredibly complex. Look at modern medicines, for example. Even though we possess today some incredibly sophisticated drugs, created at the molecular level, there is still no drug available that doesn't have some undesirable side-effect or knock-on consequence. Compare this to a natural body hormone, which works in perfect balance with all the other chemicals that exist in the body, without side effects, and you'll see my point.

246

This is why I believe that a holistic approach to looking after our bodies will ultimately prove the best option. Natural remedies, scientifically-created drugs, skilled surgery, mental health and relaxation, good diet – all of these factors play an immensely important role in our physical welfare and *all* need to be looked at in order to obtain a good solution to our health problems.

It would be wonderfully easy if we could swallow one little pill to cure an illness for good, but unfortunately for those of us who like it simple, life is not like that. This is why you – the patient – need to focus on all aspects of your illness and body, and treat yourself using any methods you find appropriate. Eat well, rest, investigate the alternatives, take medical advice, do it all. *You have more choice than you realize.* Don't let doctors tell you that complementary or dietary therapies are rubbish; but similarly, never let an alternative practitioner persuade you to reject a more proven medical treatment in favour of his or her favoured therapy, no matter how in vogue it may be. *It is your health, your body and you are the boss.* Do the research, take the best odds and remember that various treatments can work successfully hand in hand. They don't necessarily have to be mutually exclusive.

Probiotics – Bugging Us Back to Health?

One area of great interest and one which I believe will come increasingly to the fore in the battle for good gut health is the use of probiotics – that is, feeding our guts with healthy bacteria that work with our bodies to enhance not only the digestive process, but also the immune system, our energy levels and general health.

It's not new stuff: people have been drinking soured milk and yoghurt cultures for nearly 2,000 years. They've been known for their ability to confer longevity on the people that use them regularly – like the Bulgarian peasants the scientist Metchnikoff referred to in his work at the Pasteur Institute in Paris in the early 1900s.

There are hundreds, if not thousands, of strains of bacteria that inhabit the intestines. The average woman has the equivalent of about eight apples' worth (800g) of bacteria in her large bowel. Men have about 1 kilo. There are more bacteria in the intestine than there are cells in the human body. They colonize the large bowel because the gut contents slow down dramatically when they reach the colon, and because the acidity levels are lower and more favourable to bacteria in this portion of the gut.

The bacteria that populate our guts include the potentially harmful (pathogenic) strains like *E. coli* as well as the generally friendly (or 'probiotic') *bifidobacteria* and *lactobacilli*. Good bacteria help our bodies in many ways. Professor Glenn Gibson explains, '*Bifidobacteria*, for example, produce very powerful peptides (protein fragments) that inhibit food poisoning bacteria. *Lactobacilli* produce similar antimicrobials and all probiotics produce lactic acid, which inhibits pathogens because it makes the gut pH more acid – which is what gut pathogens hate. And all probiotics stimulate the immune system.'

Bifidobacteria also produce B-vitamins, and *B. longum* is able to manufacture riboflavin (vitamin B12), pyridoxine (B6), cobalamin (B12) and also vitamin C.

Normally there is a balance of bacteria, but many things can happen to skew the balance: a bout of diarrhoea, a course of broad-spectrum antibiotics, anaesthetics, stress, even diet – all these can disturb the fine balance of gut flora. Sometimes this means that the bad bugs take over, leaving the good ones in the helpless minority. Clearly, if our guts can be overrun with bad bugs, it makes sense to try and put as many good ones back in as we can. The potential benefits of populating our guts with probiotics include:

- A reduction in wind and bloating – studies show that probiotics can reduce gas formation within the bowel, which can minimize bloating and the abdominal discomfort that accompanies it.
- Increased resistance to food poisoning and infections of the gastrointestinal tract.
- Research finds that they can prevent diarrhoea associated with antibiotic treatment and infection with *Clostridium difficile*.
- Reduction in blood lipid (cholesterol) levels.
- Improved lactose tolerance.
- Improvements in healing of lesions and inflammation in the gut walls.
- A boost to the immune system. According to the Royal Free and University College Medical School's Professor Jeremy Hamilton Miller, the 'passage of small numbers of bacteria across the gut wall into the circulation (have) an immuno–stimulatory effect.' They also produce substances 'that contribute

toward the natural defences of the body, such as IgA, interferon gamma and interleukins'.

- Finnish research has shown that childhood eczema and connected allergies were 50 per cent less likely to occur in susceptible children if the mother took probiotics before the infant's birth and while breastfeeding.
- Anti-cancer properties – Japanese research has indicated a significant reduction in bladder cancer among patients regularly taking probiotic fermented milk drinks.

Does It Have What It Says on the Label?

Even though the concept of probiotics has much to commend it, putting it into practice is another issue. According to Professor Glenn Gibson, who has conducted research into probiotics products at Reading University, there is a key question that needs answering in relation to every probiotics food supplement: 'Does the product contain the strains of bacteria it claims to, and in the quantities that it states?'

The answer, unfortunately, is not always. 'Our ongoing work has shown that something like 50 per cent of current products do not match up with their labels in terms of microbial content and/or numbers of strains contained in them. Some products do not label their contents and, in certain cases, some of these do not even contain microbes actually recognized as probiotics.' However, many popular probiotic products tested by Professor Gibson have been found to contain what they claim on their labels. They include:

- ProViva, a fruit drink made by Skanemejerier that contains *L. plantarum*
- Multibionta, a multivitamin tablet with enterically-coated probiotics made by Seven Seas Health Care Ltd (UK) that contains *L. acidophilus, B. bifidum* and *B. longum*
- Benecol, a yoghurt made by Johnson & Johnson, (US) that contains bifidobacterium
- Yakult®, a fermented milk drink made by Yakult (Japan) that contains *L. casei Shirota*
- Bio Danone, a yoghurt made by Danone (France) that contains *Bifidus essensis*

- Actimel®, a fermented milk drink made by Danone (France) that contains *L. casei immunitass*

Professor Gibson believes that 'to be any good, a probiotic supplement needs to contain a bacterial count of 10^6, and the product should also provide back-up information. Many of the larger manufacturers have helplines for consumers, which are useful. This is such an important area of supplementary healthcare because so many people have gut problems, and guidelines should be set up. Probiotics are sold (in the UK) as functional foods, and so far there are only voluntary guidelines.'

Prebiotics

While probiotics are the good flora that help inhibit food poisoning, *prebiotics* are the foods that they thrive on. These foods enable the good flora to flourish in our guts and keep the balance of good versus bad bacteria tipped the right way. Prebiotics include supplements like FOS (fructooligosaccharides), GOS (Gluco-oligosaccharides) and lactulose. Good dietary sources of FOS include bananas, leeks, onions, garlic, chicory, artichoke and asparagus. And, according to Richard Palframan, Anne McCartney and Glenn Gibson, 'breast milk contains a "bifidus" factor – a glycoprotein that stimulates the growth of bifidobacteria' in the newborn infant.

A Resource Tool – Self-Help and Other Associations, Websites and Further Information

I've made every effort to print the most current addresses, telephone numbers and web-links throughout this book, but these can and do change, often more than we'd like. It's frustrating for you, and equally for me, as I want you to have the best information possible. Here's a tip: if a web address no longer works, type the name of the organization (or the disease you're researching) into the box of a good search engine like Google, and you may find links to a website that way. Always put as much relevant information into a search engine as you can – perhaps include the country, or even key words that relate to what the organization does.

General Digestive Associations

UK

Digestive Disorders Foundation, 3 St Andrew's Place, Regents Park, London NW1 4LB Tel: 020 7486 0341 Website: www.digestivedisorders.org.uk E-mail: dds@digestivedisorders.org.uk

British Society of Gastroenterology, 3 St Andrew's Place, London NW1 4LB Tel: 020 7387 3534 Website: www.bsg.org.uk E-mail: bsg@mailbox.ulcc.ac.uk

Association of Coloproctology of Great Britain and Ireland at the Royal College of Surgeons of England, 35–43 Lincoln's Inn Fields, London WC2A 3PE Tel: 020 7973 0307 Website: www.acpgbi.org.uk E-mail: acpgbi@asgbi.org.uk

US

International Foundation for Functional Gastrointestinal Disorders (IFFGD), PO Box 170864, Milwaukee, WI 53217-8076 Tel: (1) 414 964 1799 Website: www.iffgd.org and www.aboutincontinence.org E-mail: iffgd@iffgd.org

American Society of Colon & Rectal Surgeons, 85 W. Algonquin Rd., Suite 550, Arlington Heights, IL 60005 Tel: (1) 847 290 9184 Website: www.fascrs.org E-mail: ascrs@fascrs.org

The American Gastroenterological Association, 7910 Woodmont Avenue, 7th Floor, Bethesda, MD 20814 Tel: (1) 301 654 2055 Website: www.gastro.org E-mail: webinfo@gastro.org

Food Allergies

UK

Anaphylaxis Campaign, PO Box 275, Farnborough, Hampshire GU14 6SX Tel: 01252 542029 Website: www.anaphylaxis.org.uk

The British Allergy Foundation (Allergy UK), Deepdene House, 30 Bellegrove Road, Welling, Kent DA16 3PY Tel: 020 8303 8583 Website: www.allergyfoundation.com

British Society for Allergy and Environmental Medicine, PO Box 7, Knighton, Powys LD7 1WF Website: www.bsaenm.org Information: 0906 3020010 (Premium line)

Action Against Allergy (AAA), PO Box 278, Twickenham, Middlesex TW1 4QQ Tel: 020 8892 2711 Website: http://home.freeuk.com/allergyaction

US

American Academy of Allergy, Asthma and Immunology, 611 East Wells Street, Milwaukee, WI 53202 Tel: (1) 414 272 6071 Patient Information Line: (1) 800 822 2762 Website: www.aaaai.org E-mail: info@aaaai.org

The Food Allergy & Anaphylaxis Network, 10400 Eaton Place, Suite 107, Fairfax, VA 22030–2208 Tel: (1) 800 929 4040 Website: www.foodallergy.org
E-mail: faan@foodallergy.org

FURTHER READING

Zellerbach, Merla. *The Allergy Sourcebook*, Lowell House, 1998

Nutrition

UK

The British Nutrition Foundation, High Holborn House, 52–54 High Holborn, London WC1V 6RQ Tel: 020 7404 6504
Website: www.nutrition.org.uk E-mail: postbox@nutrition.org.uk

British Dietetic Association, Fifth Floor, Charles House, 148/9 Great Charles Street, Queensway, Birmingham B3 3HT Tel: 0121 200 8080 Fax: 0121 200 8081 Website: www.bda.uk.com E-mail: info@bda.uk.com

Women's Nutritional Advisory Service, PO Box 268, Lewes, East Sussex, BN7 1QN Tel: 01273 487366 Website: www.wnas.org.uk

US & CANADA

American Dietetic Association, 216 W. Jackson Blvd., Chicago, IL 60606–6995 Tel: (1) 312 899 0040 Website: www.eatright.org

The Oley Foundation (for people on parenteral/enteral nutrition), 214 Hun Memorial, A-28 Albany Medical Center, Albany, NY 12208–3478
Tel: (1) 800 776 6539 Website: www.oley.org or http://c4isr.com/oley/
E-mail: bishopj@mail.amc.edu

National Institute of Nutrition, 408 Queen Street, 3rd Floor, Ottawa, Ontario, Cananda K1R 5A7 Tel: (1) 613 235 3355
Website: www.nin.ca E-mail: nin@nin.ca

FURTHER READING

Jonsson, Gudrun. *Gut Reaction*, Random House, 1999

Coeliac Disease

UK

The Coeliac Society, PO Box 220, High Wycombe, Bucks HP11 2HY
Helpline: 0870 444 8804 Fax: 01494 474349 Website: www.coeliac.co.uk
E-mail: diet@coeliac.co.uk

US & CANADA

Celiac Disease Foundation, 13251 Ventura Boulevard, Suite 1, Studio City,
California, 91604–1838 Tel: (1) 818 990 2354 Website: www.celiac.org

Celiac Sprue Association, CSA/USA Inc., PO Box 31700, Omaha NE 68131–
0700 Website: www.csaceliacs.org E-mail: celiacs@csaceliacs.org

Gluten Intolerance Group North America, 15110 – 10th Ave SW, Suite A,
Seattle, Washington State WA 98166–1820 Website: www.gluten.net

The American Celiac Society, 59 Crystal Avenue, West Orange, New Jersey, NJ
07052 Tel: (1) 973-325-8837

Canadian Celiac Association, 5170 Dixie Road, Suite 204, Mississauga,
Ontario, L4W 1E3, Canada Website: www.celiac.ca

AUSTRALIA & NEW ZEALAND

The Coeliac Society of Australia Website: www.coeliac.org.au
(This website gives details of state society members)

Coeliac Society of New Zealand (Inc), PO Box 739 Avondale, Auckland, New
Zealand Website: www.coeliac.co.nz

FURTHER READING

Holmes, Geoffrey and Catassi, Carlo. *Fast Facts: Coeliac Disease*, Health Press,
1999

Diverticular Disease

UK

The National Association for Diverticular Disease,
7 Cambridge Road, Orrell, Wigan WN5 8PI. Helpline: (4 p.m.–7 p.m.): 01942
213572 Website: www.ukselfhelp.info/groupNADD.htm

FURTHER READING

Trickett, Shirley. *Irritable Bowel Syndrome and Diverticulosis*, Thorsons, 1999

Irritable Bowel Syndrome

UK

IBS Network, Northern General Hospital, Sheffield S5 7AU Helpline: 01543
492192 Website: www.ibsnetwork.org.uk

Irritable Bowel Syndrome Network, St John's House, Hither Green Hospital,
Hither Green Lane, London SE13 6RU Helpline: 020 8698 4611 ext 8194

US & CANADA

IBS Self Help Group, 3324 Yonge Street, PO Box 94074, Toronto, Ontario, M4N
3R1 Canada Tel: (1) 416 932 3311

AUSTRALIA

Irritable Bowel Information & Support Association of Australia Inc (IBIS), PO
Box 5044, Manly, Brisbane, Queensland, Australia 4179 Tel: (07) 3893-1131
Website: www.ibis-australia.org

FURTHER READING

Brewer, Dr Sarah and Berriedale-Johnson, Michelle. *Eat to Beat IBS*, Thorsons,
2002
Sinclair, Carol with Stewart, Dr Alan. *The IBS Starch-free Diet*, Vermilion, 1997
Trickett, Shirley. *Irritable Bowel Syndrome and Diverticulosis*, Thorsons, 1999
Hunter, Dr John; Workman, Elizabeth and Woolner, Jenny. *The New Allergy
Diet*, Vermilion, 2000

Ulcerative Colitis and Crohn's Disease

UK

Crohn's in Childhood Research Association, Parkgate House, 356 West Barnes Lane, Motspur Park, Surrey KT3 6NB   Tel: 020 8949 6209 Website: www.cicra.org   E-mail: support@cicra.org

National Association for Colitis and Crohn's Disease (NACC), 4 Beaumont House, Sutton Road, St Albans, Herts AL1 5HH   Helpline: 01727 844296 and 0845 1302233   Website: www.nacc.org.uk E-mail: nacc@nacc.org.uk

ibd Club, 6th Floor, The Tower Building, 11 York Road, London SE1 7NX   Tel: 020 7401 4080   Website: www.ibdclub.org.uk

AUSTRALIA & NEW ZEALAND

Australian Crohn's and Colitis Association, PO Box 201, Mooroolbark, Victoria 3138, Australia Tel: 1 800 138 029   Website: www.acca.net.au

Crohn's & Colitis Support Groups, PO Box 24-171, Royal Oak, Auckland, NZ Tel: 09 636 7228 or toll-free in NZ: 0508 227469 Website: www.ccsg.org.nz E-mail: ccsg@clear.net.nz

US & CANADA

The Crohn's and Colitis Foundation of America (CCFA), National Headquarters, 386 Park Avenue South, 17th Floor, New York, NY 10016 8804 Tel: (1) 800 932 2423 or (1) 212 685 3440 Website: www.ccfa.org E-mail: info@ccfa.org

Intestinal Disease Foundation, Landmarks Building, Suite 525, One Station Square, Pittsburgh, PA 15219–1138   Tel: (1) 412 261 5888   Website: www.intestinalfoundation.org

Crohn's and Colitis Foundation of Canada (CCFC), 21 St Clair Avenue East, Suite 600, Toronto, Ontario M4T 1N5   Tel: (1) 416 920 5035   Website: www.ccfc.ca

FURTHER READING

Sklar, Jill and Sklar, Manuel. *The First Year – Crohn's Disease and Ulcerative Colitis: An Essential Guide for the Newly-Diagnosed*, Marlow & Company, 2002

Digestive Cancers

UK

Cancer BACUP, 3 Bath Place, Rivington Street, London EC2A 3JR
Helpline Tel: 0808 800 1234 Website: www.cancerbacup.org.uk
E-mail: info@cancerbacup.org.uk

Cancer Research UK, 61 Lincoln's Inn Fields, London WC2A 3PX
Tel: 020 7242 0200 Website: www.cancer.org.uk

Colon Cancer Concern, 9 Rickett Street, London SW6 1RU Infoline: 08708 506050 (Mon-Fri 10a.m.–4p.m., 24-hr answerphone)
Website: www.coloncancer.org.uk E-mail: info@coloncancer.org.uk

Oesophageal Patients Association, 16 Whitefields Crescent, Solihull, West Midlands B91 3NU Helpline: 0121 704 9860 Website: www.opa.org.uk

US & CANADA

American Cancer Society, Website: www.cancer.org

Oncolink, Website: http://cancer.med.upenn.edu

Canadian Cancer Society, National Office, Suite 200, 10 Alcorn Avenue, Toronto, Ontario, M4V 3B1 Tel: (1) 888 939 3333 Website: www.cancer.ca
E-mail: info@cis.cancer.ca

AUSTRALIA & NEW ZEALAND

The Cancer Council Australia, GPO Box 4708, Sydney, NSW 2001,
Level 5, Medical Foundation Building, 92–94 Paramatta Rd, Camperdown NSW 2050 Tel: 61 2 9036 3100
Website: www.cancer.org.au E-mail: info@cancer.org.au

Cancer Society of New Zealand Inc., PO Box 10847, Wellington   Website: www.cancernz.org.nz E-mail: admin@cancernz.org.nz

EUROPE

Cancereurope, Website: www.cancerworld.org

FURTHER READING

Understanding Cancer of the Stomach, published by CancerBACUP, 2001

Understanding Cancer of the Large Bowel (Colon and rectum), published by CancerBACUP, 2001

Young, Annie M. (editor) et al. *ABC of Colorectal Cancer*, BMJ Books, 2001

Ostomy Associations

UK

The Ileostomy and Internal Pouch Support Group (ia), Peverill House, 1–5 Mill Road, Ballyclare, Co. Antrim BT39 9DR Helpline: 0800 0184724 Website: www.ileostomypouch.demon.co.uk

Pouch Care Nurse, Red Lion Group (for internal pouch owners), St Mark's Hospital, Northwick Park, Watford, Harrow HA1 3UJ Tel: 0208 235 4126 Website: http://ourworld.compuserve.com/homepages/timrogers/redliong.htm

British Colostomy Association, 15 Station Road, Reading, Berkshire RG1 1LG Freephone: 0800 328 4257 Website: www.bcass.org.uk E-mail: sue@bcass.org.uk

Coloplast Limited, Peterborough Business Park, Peterborough, PE2 6FX Tel: 01733 392000 Website: www.coloplast.co.uk

Convatec Limited, Harrington House, Milton Road, Ickenham, Uxbridge UB10 8PU Helpline: 0800 282254 Website: www.convatec.com

Dansac Limited, Victoria House, Vision Park, Histon, Cambridge CB4 5JD Tel: 01223 235100 Website: www.dansac.co.uk

Gay Ostomates Association, (Syd McCaffrey, secretary), 72 Tramway Road, Aigburth, Liverpool L17 7AZ Tel: 0151 726 9019
Website: http://freespace.virgin.net/alan.edinburgh/goa.html
E-mail: sydmccaffrey.goa@bushinternet.com

US & CANADA

United Ostomy Association (UCA), 19772 MacArthur Blvd, Suite 200, Irvine, CA 92612-2405   Tel: (1) 800 826 0826 Website: www.uoa.org
E-mail: info@uoa.org

Wound, Ostomy & Continence Nurses Society (WOCN), 4700 W. Lake Ave, Glenview IL 60025   Tel: (1) 888 224 WOCN (toll free) or (1) 866 615 8560
Website: www.wocn.org

INTERNATIONAL

International Ostomy Association, Website: www.ostomyinternational.org

FURTHER READING

Dorr Muller, Barbara and McGinn, Kerr Anne. *The Ostomy Book – Living Comfortably with Colostomies, Ileostomies and Urostomies*, Bull Publishing, 1992

Continence

UK

The Helpline Nurse, The Continence Foundation (Incontinence Information Helpline), 307 Hatton Square, 16 Baldwins Gardens, London EC1N 7RJ Helpline: 0845 345 0165 (Mon–Fri 9.30a.m.–12-30p.m.)
Website: www.continence-foundation.org.uk
E-mail: continence-help@ dial.pipex.com

Incontact, United House, North Road, London N7 9DP Helpline: 0870 770 3246 Website: www.incontact.org E-mail: info@incontact.org

Association for Continence Advice (ACA), 102a Astra House, Arklow Road, New Cross, London SE14 6EB Tel: 020 8692 4680 Website: www.aca.uk.com
E-mail: info@aca.uk.com

US & CANADA

The Simon Foundation for Continence, PO Box 835, Wilmette, Illinois 60091   Tel: (1) 800 23 SIMON (toll free) or (1) 847 864 3913   Website: www.simonfoundation.org

National Association for Continence, PO Box 8310, Spartanburg, SC 29305–8310   Tel: (1) 864 579 7900 Website: www.nafc.org
E-mail: memberservices@nafc.org

The Canadian Continence Foundation, PO Box 30, Victoria Branch, Westmount, Qc. H3Z 2V4 Consumer Helpline: (1) 800 265 9575 Website: www.continence-fdn.ca   E-mail: help@continence-fdn.ca

AUSTRALIA & NEW ZEALAND

Continence Foundation of Australia Ltd, AMA House, 293 Royal Parade, Parkville, Victoria 3052 Helpline: 1 800 330066 Website: www.contfound.org.au
E-mail: info@contfound.org.au

New Zealand Continence Association Inc., PO Box 270, Drury 1750 Helpline: 0800 650 659   Website: www.continence.org.nz   E-mail: jan@continence.org.nz

Sexuality

UK

Association to aid the Sexual and Personal Relationships of People with a Disability (SPOD), 286 Camden Road, London, N7 0BJ Helpline Tel: 020 7607 8851   Website: www.spod-uk.org E-mail: info@spod-uk.org

British Association for Sexual and Relationship Therapy, PO Box 13686, London SW20 9ZH Tel: 020 8543 2707 Website: www.basmt.org.uk
E-mail: info@basrt.org.uk

FURTHER READING

Morin, Ph.D, Jack. *Anal Pleasure & Health – A Guide for Men and Women*, Down There Press, 1998

Travel

UK

Medical Advisory Services for Travellers Abroad (MASTA), 52 Margaret Street, London W1W 8SQ

Traveller's Health Line: 0906 822 4100 (Premium rate)   Website: www.masta.org.uk

Medicines and Medical Support

UK

Medicines Control Agency (MCA), Market Towers, 1 Nine Elms Lane, London SW8 5NQ Tel: 020 7273 0000 Website: www.mca.gov.uk/ E-mail: info@mca.gsi.gov.uk

Steroid Aid Group, PO Box 220, London E17 3JR

Group Against Steroid Prescriptions (GASP), 70–72 Costa Street, South Bank, Middlesbrough, North Yorkshire TS6 6EU Helpline: 01642 465118

Medic Alert Foundation, 1 Bridge Wharf, 156 Caledonian Road, London N1 9UU Tel: 020 7833 3034 Website: www.medicalert.co.uk E-mail: info@medicalert.co.uk (For medical talisman bracelets and necklaces)

RADAR, 12 City Forum, 250 City Road, London EC1V 8AF Tel: 020 7250 3222 Website: www.radar.org.uk (For keys to approx. 4,000 locked public toilets in and around the UK)

US & CANADA

The MedicAlert Foundation USA, 2323 Colorado Avenue, Turlock, CA 95382–2018 Tel: (1) 888 633 4298 Website: www.medicalert.org

RxList (Internet drug Index), Website: www.rxlist.com E-mail: info@rxlist.com

Medicare Website: www.medicare.gov

The MedicAlert Foundation Canada, 2005 Sheppard Ave East, Suite 800, Toronto, Ontario M2J 5B4 Tel: (1) 800 668 1507 Website: www.medicalert.ca

AUSTRALIA & NEW ZEALAND

The MedicAlert Foundation Australia, 216 Greenhill Road, Eastwood, South Australia 5063 Tel: 1 800 88 22 22   Website: www.medicalert.com.au

The MedicAlert Foundation New Zealand, PO Box 40028, Astral Towers, Main Street, Upper Hutt 6007 New Zealand Tel: 64 4 528 8219
Website: www.medicalert.co.nz   E-mail: medicalert@clear.net.nz

FURTHER READING

Henry, Professor John A. *The British Medical Association New Guide to Medicines and Drugs*, Dorling Kindersley, 2001
Rybacki, Pharm.D., James. *The Essential Guide to Prescription Drugs 2002*, HarperCollins, 2001

Government Agencies

UK

Department of Health, Richmond House, 79 Whitehall, London SW1A 2NS Tel: 020 7210 4850 Website: www.doh.gov.uk

Health Development Agency, Holborn Gate, 330 High Holborn, London WC1V 7BA Tel: 020 7430 0850   Website: www.hda-online.org.uk

US

National Institutes of Health, Bethesda, Maryland, 20892   Tel: (1) 301 496 4000   Website: www.nih.gov

National Institute of Diabetes and Digestive and Kidney Diseases, NIH, Building 31, Room 9A04 Center Drive, MSC 2560, Bethesda, MD 20892-2560 Website: www.niddk.nih.gov/   E-mail: niddc@info.niddk.nih.gov

Centers for Disease Control and Prevention, 1600 Clifton Road, Atlanta, GA 30333   Tel: (1) 800 311 3435   Website: www.cdc.gov

Food and Drug Administration (FDA), 5600 Fishers Lane, Rockville, MD 20857
Tel: (1) 888 463 6332   Website: www.fda.gov

INTERNATIONAL

World Health Organisation. Website: www.who.int

Complementary Therapies

UK

British Medical Acupuncture Society, 12 Marbury House, Higher Whitley,
Warrington, Cheshire WA4 4QW Tel: 01925 730727
Website: www.medical-acupuncture.co.uk

UK Homeopathic Medical Association, 6 Livingstone Road, Gravesend, Kent
DA12 5DZ Tel: 01474 560336   Website: www.homoeopathy.org

British Homeopathic Association (BHA), 15 Clerkenwell Close, London EC1R
0AA   Tel: 020 7566 7800   Website: www.trusthomeopathy.org

US & CANADA

American Academy of Medical Acupuncture (AAMA), 4929 Wilshire
Boulevard, Suite 428, Los Angeles, California 90010 Tel: (1) 323 937 5514
Website: www.medicalacupuncture.org E-mail: JDOWDEN@prodigy.net

American Institute of Homeopathy, 801 N. Fairfax Street, Suite 306,
Alexandria, Virginia 22314 Tel: (1) 888 445 9988
Website: www.homeopathyusa.org E-mail: aih@homeopathyusa.org

Acupuncture Foundation of Canada Institute (AFCI), 2131 Lawrence Avenue
East, Ste 204, Scarborough, Ontario M1R 5G4 Canada Tel: (1) 416 752 3988
Website: www.afcinstitute.com E-mail: info@afcinstitute.com

Homeopathic Medical Council of Canada, 3910 Bathurst Street, Suite 202,
Toronto, Ontario, Canada M3H 3N8 Tel: (1) 416 638 4622
Website: www.hmcc.ca E-mail: info@hmcc.ca

AUSTRALIA & NEW ZEALAND

Australian Homeopathic Association

Tel: 08 8346 3961 (Secretary Sue McCormick)

Website: www.homeopathyoz.org   E-mail: smick@smartchat.net.au

FURTHER READING

Shealy, Norman C. *The Illustrated Encyclopaedia of Healing Remedies*, Element, 1998

Westwood, Christine. *Aromatherapy – A Guide for Home Use*, Amberwood Publishing, 1991

If you have any comments about any of the information mentioned in this book or would like to suggest other useful organizations or weblinks, please contact me at the following address:

Stephanie Zinser
c/o Thorsons
HarperCollins*Publishers*
77–85 Fulham Palace Road
Hammersmith
London W6 8JB

Index

abdomen 8, 22–4, 39, 64
    pain 71, 75, 90, 94, 201
    surgery 211–17
    X-rays 45
abscesses
    anal 23, 25, 134–5
    intra-abdominal 216
acetylsalicylic acid 63
acupuncture 50
Addenbrooke's NHS Trust
    138
additives 76
adhesions 23, 123–5
adrenaline 57
aerophagy 26
AfraidToAsk.com 95
agendas 38
airtight underwear 28
alcohol 13, 17, 23, 30, 55–7
allergies 75–81, 85–9, 200,
    252
alternative therapies 50–1
Altruis Biomedical Network
    18
aluminium 65
American Academy of
    Paediatrics 207
American Cancer Society
    197
American Dietic
    Association 84
American Society of Colon
    and Rectal Surgeons
    135
American Thyroid
    Association 105
amoebiasis 112–14
amoebic dysentary 112–14
amylase 4, 5

anaphylaxis 76, 77–8, 79,
    80
anastomosis 213, 217, 218
anatomy 3–7
Anti-Parasite.com 113, 118
antibiotics 13, 16, 55, 62–3
antidepressants 65
antigens 47
anus 6–7, 34, 41
    abscesses 23, 25, 134–5
    cancer 19, 21, 25, 29,
      197–9
    fissures 19, 25, 31, 70,
      137–8, 200
    fistulas 19, 21, 25, 135–6
    intercourse 21, 38
    sphincter 5, 7, 43
appendicitis 14, 16, 23,
    180–2, 200, 202
appendix 6–7
appetite 40
aromatherapy 50
aspirin 23, 64–5
asthmatics 76
athlete's diarrhoea 59–60
Ayurveda 32

babies 14, 21, 24, 31, 78, 83
back passage 8, 25–6, 35
bacteria 7, 16, 26–7, 41
    food poisoning 108–10,
      114
    nutrition 78
barium
    enemas 45–7
    meal 45
    swallow 45
bars 9
beans 10, 26

Beating Bowel Cancer 194
beauty regime 69
belching 34
bidets 25
Bifidobacterium longum
    16, 26, 63, 95, 248
bile 5
bleeding 18–20, 39
    aspirin 64
    back passage 8
    checklist 39
    false 72–3
    gastrointestinal 47
bloating 26–8, 71, 75, 81
blockages 183–4
blood 8, 33, 84
    sugar 71
    tests 42–3
body image 228, 242
bone chemistry 43
bone densitometry (DEXA)
    scan 45
botulism 9, 16, 118–19
bowels 7, 9, 14, 18–19
    cancer 23, 29, 47
    control 29
    mucus 21
    opening 35
    perforation 51
    pouches 71
    problems 33
    symptoms 48
    tumours 27
breast cancer 7, 33
breath tests 42
British Allergy Foundation
    76, 79, 80, 84
British Diabetic Association
    74

266